What If...?

Finding new adventures through life's obstacles

ROBERTA E. SAWATZKY

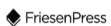

One Printers Way
Altona, MB R0G 0B0
Canada

www.friesenpress.com

Copyright © 2023 by Roberta E. Sawatzky, MA, GPHR
First Edition — 2023

All rights reserved.

No part of this publication may be reproduced in any form, or by any means, electronic or mechanical, including photocopying, recording, or any information browsing, storage, or retrieval system, without permission in writing from FriesenPress.

ISBN
978-1-03-917756-7 (Hardcover)
978-1-03-917755-0 (Paperback)
978-1-03-917757-4 (eBook)

1. BIOGRAPHY & AUTOBIOGRAPHY, PERSONAL MEMOIRS

Distributed to the trade by The Ingram Book Company

TESTIMONIALS

"All the stages of life incorporate our experiences which propel us forward in new directions. Why should it be any different for the transition to our retirement stage or change to our working structures? And yet, we start "down-sizing" our dreams and opportunities. Roberta Sawatzky has written a book that challenges these parameters. She shares her stories and how they inform new ways of thinking and being. We all are growing and contributing individuals and this book charts a course beginning with where we come from to the possibilities in front of us. I found Sawatzky to be a masterful storyteller as she weaves her life and perspectives into a book that challenged me to rethink both my travel and livelihood."

—C. Fast, Freelance Business Consultant

"*What If...*' captivated me. The refreshing honesty with which the author painted the picture of life with its rollercoaster resonated deeply. Incorporating the story of a family's journey with kidney disease, coupled with the empowering message of choice and resilience, left me thoroughly inspired."

—T. Atkinson, Kidney Foundation of Canada

"This compelling narrative of celebration and challenge; of honest, authentic and sometimes raw emotion inspires and encourages the reader to take chances. I loved being reminded to approach our retirement years with the same optimism, sense of adventure and recklessness as we did in our early years - to approach obstacles practically but, more importantly with positive intent and deliberation.

A great read applicable to all seasons of life's journey. *What if…? Why not…!"*

—C. COLPITTS, PERFORMER, PRODUCER, ARRANGER, & TRAVELLER

"Everyone has at some point asked themselves a big '*What if..?'* question. For those who have been bold enough to embrace the answer, Roberta's words will transport you back to that moment. The excitement, the challenges, the reactions of others, and those moments of discovery when the world slows down and you experience something brand new with fresh eyes. The magical happenings only granted to those who step outside their comfortable groove. And for those pondering the question, you need this book even more. Whatever your life stage or background, travel has that power to reveal hidden facets of your own self, and your relationships, as you see new sides of the world. Sharing Roberta's journey will help you to shape your own adventures, and celebrate every life-changing memory they create."

—M. MIDDLEMISS, FREELANCE AUTHOR AND JOURNALIST

The deepest satisfaction of writing is precisely that it opens up new spaces within us of which we were not aware before we started to write. To write is to embark on a journey whose final destination we do not know.

—Henri Nouwen

WWW.HENRINOUWEN.ORG

INTRODUCTION

Retirement is not the end of the road.
It is the beginning of the open highway.

—U<small>NKNOWN</small>

"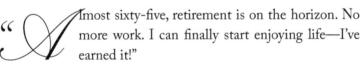lmost sixty-five, retirement is on the horizon. No more work. I can finally start enjoying life—I've earned it!"

How many times had I heard that sentiment? People look forward to having an abundance of discretionary time on their hands to do…what? Many don't have hobbies but are filled with dreams of taking up golf, travelling more, or finally learning to cook those amazing, mouth-watering dishes prepared by home chefs who somehow just know how to cook in banana leaves or bake a perfect croquembouche. Others dream of finally learning how to dance, moving to a log house by a babbling brook, or another special something they have been putting off for retirement. To many, Freedom 65 means having more time with family and friends, recycling work clothes, escaping cold winters in favour of a palm-tree-lined Malecon and umbrella drinks. However, before too long, boredom sets in. The excitement of anticipated freedom fades, the expected thrill of new endeavours is found to be overrated, and travel on a budget lacks a certain appeal. Days turn to weeks, weeks to months, and before long, the first-year anniversary of retirement arrives, along with the realisation that something is missing—purpose.

As I observed these scenarios in other's lives, I knew I wanted something different, something that didn't mark the end of a purpose-filled career, but rather the beginning of what might be a new found purpose. I had just turned sixty-one.

As such a life transition looms before those of us in the Jones Generation (born between 1954 and 1965), many of us are pausing to ask, is the only choice to work or retire? What if we can't afford to retire? Do we enter this chapter discouraged and browbeaten, because life has not afforded us the wherewithal to build a nest egg? Are we doomed to work until our bodies and minds simply can't produce anymore? How depressing! Does an alternative exist? Can we leave the craziness of a nine-to-five workday while not abandoning it altogether? Can we take time to enjoy the fruits of our labour while not falling prey to a life of self-servitude?

People of all ages need to know they are valuable contributors; for many of us, that comes through the work we do and the active roles we play in our communities. I don't ever want to become redundant or stop challenging old ideas, contributing new ones, and influencing others to persist, making a difference wherever I go, whatever I do.

Society tells us we deserve to retire at sixty-five to a life filled with travel and leisure; however, I want to encourage a change in mindset. Imagine it's your fifty-fifth birthday and you are blowing out a staggering number of candles on your cake. Your family and friends all begin chanting, "Make a wish, make a wish!" Immediately, your mind thinks about the conversation you had with your advisor the previous week. Your wish? In ten years, you hope you can afford to retire from the routine and demands of a schedule dictated by someone else. You want to be free!

Not too many people could find fault with such a wish. However, what if you tweaked it a little? What if finding freedom meant more than the exit from regular work and the loss of a monthly income? What if freedom involved embracing opportunities to earn an income on your own terms? What if your wish included a ten-year plan that would see you transitioning, not retiring, to a purpose-filled endeavour that would draw on your experience, knowledge, and wisdom? What if there were more options than simply retiring? How remarkable to keep contributing to organisations, younger generations, families, friends, and communities, on your own terms?

I have confidence in this as a better option. My desire is that when you close this book, you will stop, reflect, and consider the idea that moving toward your retirement years does not mean you have to stop making a difference and having an impact. But rather, you can continue living a life of significant contribution to society that is not limited by lack of financial resources. Many obstacles can be placed before us at any life stage, but more so as we approach what many consider our "golden years." This book is about creatively finding ways to overcome such obstacles in order to keep doing what we love and what we're good at, and doing it in unison with how we want to continue contributing to those activities and areas we feel most passionate about.

I dearly love my family and friends, love to travel, love to learn, *and* love the work I do. I have no intention of starting counting the days until I finally have the freedom to quit work and kick back. I intend to embrace all soul filling aspects of life, following a path paved with valuable contributions, lessons, challenges—and yes, income-earning, for as long as possible.

As I looked to the future, my plan was to combine an extended study leave with international travel. Together with my husband, this experience would present the chance to engage in work that I love, create great learning opportunities, all experienced in the context of a love of travel. To be clear, this would in no way be my farewell-to-working year, rather, my way to experience what it would be like to embrace a location independent context of working. It would call on my ability to self-manage the when, where, and how of getting work done. An exciting adventure, indeed.

Let me take a moment to share a bit about me and what makes me tick. While I didn't realise it at the time, I have been working remotely in some form for the past twenty-nine years! Before I get ahead of myself, let's hit pause and clarify what I mean by "working remote." Simply put, remote working refers to those who can do their work from a location other than a physical or central office space shared with their co-workers. This shared office space would be operated by the organization they work for. Another way to put it would be *working from anywhere.*

I had the privilege of being a stay-at-home mom until our youngest child went to kindergarten. At that time I was offered a leadership role at a non-profit organisation. I was quite excited at the prospect of taking on work—and getting paid! However, I was not ready to give up on the joys of being part of my children's lives both in and out of their schooling; they were—and always will be—my priority. Did going back to work mean I had to abandon those special parenting moments?

I knew what I wanted, so before accepting, I decided to ask for the moon, in other words, I lay out some conditions: if my kids were sick, I could work from home; I could attend all scheduled field trips; and, finally, I would be able to adjust my work hours to facilitate volunteering at the school. I also offered the assurance that in no way would the quality of my work or the leadership of my teams suffer. To my surprise and delight, they agreed! That set the precedent going forward; I was never denied the privilege of such a flexible schedule, nor did I ever take it for granted. On top of all this, the organisations I worked for provided me support through time and funding to complete a Master of Arts degree in leadership, granting me the opportunity to immediately and directly apply all I was learning to my current role. I continually count my blessings for such amazing employers and leaders committed to the growth and development of their employees. And I am eternally grateful for an amazingly supportive husband who was—and is—my greatest support and cheerleader.

Unknowingly, my career experiences inspired both of our children to pursue non-traditional work. Our son embraced a six-year stint living a digital nomad lifestyle, while travelling and working in Europe (with his wife and six kids!)—and our daughter also works remotely for an organisation headquartered in the United States.

In 2008, Canada suffered a recession and jobs were being cut. I led a team responsible for developing and sourcing leadership training resources. Because we were not a revenue-generating department, we were the logical area for jobs to be cut… . I received my termination notice. After the shock wore off and the anger abated, I made the decision to start a home-based consulting business, giving birth to Sawatzky & Associates Management Consulting (SAM) in 2009. Fast forward to 2012, and in addition to my consulting business, focusing on all things remote, I joined the ranks of academia and become a business professor specialising in human resources and management. This academic involvement provided me with the access and funding to dip my toes into what, for me, were uncharted waters: research. My area of interest and passion? Remote work. My academic career continues to open doors for me to accept speaking opportunities in places like Finland, Hungary, France, and Gran Canarias, to travel for research while fulfilling my various responsibilities as a professor.

I love a challenge! That means saying yes to things before thinking through my current capacity. As a result, I have suffered burnout and been forced to pull out of activities—and even relationships—that drained me. Finding balance is a challenge when your work straddles the virtual and physical worlds. I have always endeavoured to honour my employer as well as my private consulting/coaching clients. The upside is that these challenging times remind me to focus on my strengths and pour my energies into areas where I can have the greatest impact.

People often ask where I most like to work. Well, it depends on what I'm doing. Quiet, focused work happens from my home office, creative thinking and writing happen in a coffee shop, teaching happens both virtually and face-to-face, and certain tasks of a more collaborative nature happen in my office on campus. When I think about my ideal writing environment, it is always a place that allows me to daydream. I need to be able to look out a window—or better yet, actually be outside. Throw in an ocean view and I'm good to go.

I have always gotten bored of routine—and when I get bored, my mind wanders to places I would rather be. Each day is a little different, depending on the nature of the work I need to do. On the days I teach, I build my day around class time and student meetings; in between all that, I carve out time to dedicate to my own business, when I can be found at home, in a café, or engaged in virtual meetings with colleagues and clients across the globe. To be honest, I like to think my evenings are shut-off times. However, that's not always the case—often, my work bleeds into the evening hours. But I do try to shut off by 7 p.m. One of my biggest challenges is to take time (anytime during the day) for quiet moments of reflection—and to simply breathe! Still, no matter how busy I am, if my family needs me, they get me.

As with everyone, I need community to be at my best. I have an incredibly supportive family (specifically, my husband, kids, and niece) who serve as the best support a person could ask for. They have no problem speaking truth to me when the need arises. I also have an amazing group of friends with whom I can laugh and cry, be crazy, serious, or intense—and even solve the world's problems. And I grew up in Ireland, right on the Irish Sea, so my happy place is the ocean—being there always seems to put life into perspective.

I am a passionate person who puts 100 percent into everything I believe in and care about. If I don't see the point or purpose of something, I really struggle to give it my all. I value freedom. I value purposeful work. I value making an impact. I value new experiences and learning. I can't resist challenging the status quo. I fight being put in a box, being tied to routine, and being bound by four walls. Flexible work—working from anywhere—is a great fit for me. There are times when I need to be in the office more days than I like... that's the reality of my work. However, if it continues for too long, I get really antsy, grumpy, and totally unproductive (just ask those I work with).

Since I spoke my first words, my favourite one has always been *why*? So I ask, why does all this matter? Why do I want to provide the reader with insight into who I am and what I care about? As I live through the years when most people have their eye set on retirement, I want something different. Thus, when given the opportunity to have an extended study leave, I want to use the time to learn, to explore, to experience, to wander, to be a sojourner, to have an impact, and to hopefully light a spark in the hearts and minds of others, encouraging them to step outside the expected with open arms and open minds. To choose an exciting option—to exchange the nine-to-five life for something exciting, meaningful, productive, and fulfilling. When I turned sixty, a friend gave me a card with the following on the front:

"Life should not be a journey to the grave with the intention of arriving safely in a pretty and well-preserved body, but rather to skid in broadside in a cloud of smoke, thoroughly used up, totally worn out, and loudly proclaiming, 'Wow! What a Ride!'"

—Hunter S. Thompson

CHAPTER 1

*Life can only be understood backwards;
but it must be lived forwards.*

—Soren Kierkegaard

How many people can say their dad was a pantyhose salesman? And who can say their dad was the top pantyhose salesman in the United Kingdom? I can!

I grew up in Bangor, Northern Ireland, in a stable home with parents who loved me, grandparents who loved me, and friends I simply could not survive without. I still remember the pounding of my heart as Alison, my best friend, and I penguin-walked up a 12 percent grade road in our subdivision, pushing the large rubber break of our roller skates into the flagstone footpath to keep from spiralling back down prematurely. Then came the thrill, the whole point of the climb: knees bent, hair blown back, heart racing, squealing like the fearless tomboys we were, as our roller skates carried us at superhero speed toward the fence that would serve as our ultimate break. I visited that same subdivision a few years ago and was shocked at how steep that hill actually was… no way would I have allowed my kids to do what we did!

Never a year went by without our family of five heading out

on some adventure to explore undiscovered spots in England, Scotland, the South of Ireland—and even Ibiza. Remember I said Dad was the top salesman? Well, the reward for being top salesman was an all-expense trip for the family to any location of our choosing. So my parents did the research and determined Ibiza, Spain would be our destination. It still stands out as a highlight of my childhood travels. We enjoyed walks by the Mediterranean, bullfights (yup, the real thing), shopping in Old Town, staying in a five-star hotel, and a lovely maid named Maria who faithfully brought us toilet paper (no idea why I remember that!).

And of course, we learned there was a reason for taking a siesta during the hottest time of day. You see, we thought we had made an incredible discovery—if you go to the swimming pool between noon and two in the afternoon, you have the whole place to yourself! No fighting over pool chairs, no lack of clean towels, and no sun worshippers annoyed by three Irish kids coming from the rainy Emerald Isle to lavish in the warmth of the mid-day Spanish sun. It was all good until we were getting ready for dinner when the fair pigment of our skin turned a deep red, clearly visible through the multitude of freckles, produced by our exposure to the blistering sun during a time when nobody in their right mind would be outside—not even in the shade. Apparently, being in the water does not qualify as sun protection. We survived, with the liberal application of after-sun soothers, and had another wonderful lived experience to add to our growing memories of travel.

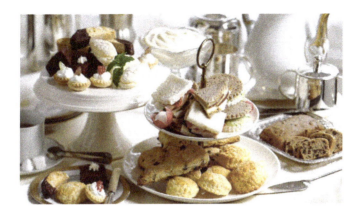

Typical afternoon tea

Travel—and feasting in great restaurants—became central to our upbringing. And we loved every experience presented. Our favourite Saturday afternoon drive always ended up at a restaurant called Winnienos (I honestly have no idea how to spell the name), often accompanied by our grandparents, Nanny and Granda McReady. I remember the spread unique to British afternoon tea. Imagine a round table, set for seven, in a bay window, filled with delicacies, as pictured above, overlooking an English garden complete with a swing hanging from a huge tree. This is where I developed a love of scones with homemade strawberry jam, topped with a dollop of fresh Devonshire cream. My mouth is watering!

Experiencing the beauty of our country was important to our family. Walking along the Irish Sea, climbing across the black rocks and finding crabs in the many tidepools, hiking the Mourne Mountains, exploring the Giant's Causeway, playing in the sand dunes at Tyrella Beach, swimming in the frigid waters of Pickie Pool, or riding a horse-drawn cart in Killarney around the Gap of Dunloe (OK, still a little bitter here—I really wanted to ride a horse, but had to ride in the cart!). Rain or shine, we took it all in.

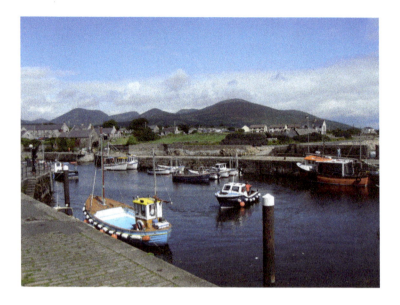

Annalong Harbour

But life in Ireland wasn't without dark shadows. If you know your UK and Irish history, you'll recall the sixties and seventies as the time of Ireland's Troubles. I remember my mum pacing, keeping a steady eye on the old clock on the mantelpiece as the hour drew near for Dad to return home from work. You see, his sales territory included such places as Belfast, Londonderry, Newry… cities that housed some of the large historic department stores like Anderson & McAuley, Robinson & Cleaver, and Sinclair's—all Dad's clients. These same cities were hot spots for the Troubles. I vividly remember a day when my Dad arrived home for dinner as pale as a ghost. He relived the horror of having walked past a bank in Belfast that was blown up not many minutes after. A man walking not far behind him wasn't so lucky.

Besides being an amazing salesman, Dad was a lay preacher. That meant on weekends, he traded in his briefcase for a Bible and passionately shared his faith at Baptist and Brethren congregations. Dad's longing for many years had been to go into full-time ministry, so after what I imagine to have been much thought and consideration, my parents informed me, my brother, and my sister that we would be totally uprooting, moving to Canada. Looking back, I know how much of a sacrifice this must have been for my parents; they left family, friends, a well-paying job, and a lovely home for a new country with no guarantee of employment (but with a much brighter future for their three children—who were two, almost twelve, and fourteen at the time of immigration).

And so, on the first of October 1970, the Campbell family touched down in Toronto, Ontario and descended the steps of a 747 British Airlines plane to begin a whole new adventure. I, for one, was pumped! Perhaps it was the excitement of new adventures, perhaps it was naïveté about the tough days to come, or perhaps it reflected my impulsiveness and readiness to try new things. No matter—I was excited!

For the first ten months, our family was physically divided; my brother and I lived with one uncle, aunt, and two cousins in their apartment in Mississauga, while our parents and sister lived with another uncle and his four kids in Oakville. Much of that time is a blur to me. Going from a primary school with maybe two hundred students to a junior high with several hundred remains a source of nightmares for me. I still recall the embarrassment of not being able to find my locker, forgetting the lock combination, and missing my classes because I couldn't find the room. Such vivid memories. Life wasn't easy, and I know my parents sheltered us from many of the hardships they faced—but we settled in, and Canada became home to us. Looking back at the life our parents created for us in this new world, I will be forever grateful. They demonstrated what it means to live courageously, to follow your passion, and be open to new experiences—an example that impacted not only me, but our children.

At the time, I really had no idea how that move would impact my life. When I look back at lessons learned, although at the time I had no clue what I was learning, I truly am grateful for the sacrifice my parents made. Arriving in big Canada from little Ireland, making new friends as a preteen, accepting charity (my father going from top salesman to pastor meant a major drop in income for our family), replacing roller skates for wobbly ice-skates on bumpy frozen lakes, walking to school in the dead of winter and having our nostrils freeze, and exploring another part of the world—all this would, without a doubt, leave its mark.

I learned that meanings differ from country to country, and that calling your Grade 6 teacher a stupid ass is not such a great idea. In Ireland, it wasn't swearing, though still disrespectful. I still remember how the teacher's face flushed to match his red hair. By the time he recovered from the shock, I was halfway home!

I learned how words have different meanings in different countries. I recall an embarrassing moment for my Dad following a lovely dinner at the home of one of his parishioners. Dad wanted to pay them a compliment and offered that they had a homely home (which is a great compliment in Ireland). All too late he realized the Canadian equivalent would be "homey", rather than homely (my poor dad!).

I learned that you are never too old—or too young—to create new friendships. After living in the Toronto area for ten months, Dad was invited to pastor a church in Bracebridge, Ontario. Right in the middle of the amazing Muskoka's. During the two years we lived there, each of us quickly built deep friendships. Hard not to do when the first winter finds you sliding off your roof right onto the snowbanks or heading out into the wild on snowmobiles with new friends, no parents, no cell phones—with the oldest among us being fourteen! Such freedom. The bonds our parents created with other parents may have been the result of shared worry over their teenagers' newfound freedom. I think that's when my mom started going grey!

I learned that not everyone who says they want to be your friend is sincere. Sometimes they just want to hear the funny way you speak. "Come skip rope with us" or "Come sit with us for lunch" weren't invitations to join the cool kids. Nope—not when you end up leaving the group close to tears as they repeat everything you say in a poor attempt at an Irish accent. Little wonder my Irish brogue faded after such a short time. But there were others, like Cheryl and Leanne, who welcomed me with open arms, funny accent and all.

I learned that you shouldn't be afraid to say yes to a challenge. Know yourself, and your strengths, and go for it. To be honest, I'm not sure where this confidence and independence came from, but throughout my life, my response to a new opportunity or challenge has always been yes. Say yes, then figure out how to do it.

I remember having chickenpox and not wanting anyone to come into my darkened room; I'd get through it on my own. Asking for help was not something I often did. And sadly, being affirmed for being *me* was also *not* part of our family's terms of endearment. So, I learned to depend on myself (not a great thing). Time passes and opportunities are presented. And guess what? The qualities I used to get in trouble for were the very qualities that equipped me to say yes to these opportunities. The key? if you don't know, ask... and keep asking.

I learned the most important learning doesn't happen within the four walls of a classroom... travel is one of the greatest teachers of all.

For example, if you get something tangled around your legs while swimming in the Mediterranean, it's not necessarily an octopus. Picture this: the water is ink-black and smooth as glass. The midday sun is beating down, and I—an eleven-year-old strong swimmer—am ready for an adventure–so why not jump into this blackness and experience something new?

All good—if your imagination is not as powerful as your curiosity. I had just finished a long walk along the sea, in the extreme heat, and relished the experience of watching fishermen catching and killing their latest catch, an octopus. It was our last day in Ibiza, and we still hadn't swum in the sea. It was time. I was only in the sea for ten minutes when it happened. I felt something—something slimy, something with bumps on it. The blackness of the water blocked my vision. It *had* to be an octopus! I screamed bloody murder as only an eleven-year-old girl could do. Finally, my Dad realizing my immense fear, dove in to rescue me. By this time, a crowd of spectators had gathered—among them, a thirteen-year-old boy who was the cutest thing ever. Puppy love does not bode well when in that position. Eventually, with Dad's help, I climbed onto the rocks, legs released from a tangled bunch of seaweed!

Needless to say, I survived, dignity shredded. However, I did learn that an overactive imagination can create deep-seated fears that eventually need to be faced.

Years later (OK, decades later), we were travelling in Italy. It was the end of a spectacular day hiking the trail joining the five villages of Cinque Terre. The black ink of the Mediterranean was every bit as lovely and intimidating as it had been decades earlier. The sweat beaded on my forehead, my legs felt like rubber, and the cure lay right in front of me. Do octopuses still live in these waters? The conversation that happened in my mind was beyond crazy. Was the reward of being completely refreshed in the cool of the Mediterranean worth the risk of encountering whatever swam below in those dark, inky waters? Fortunately, my eleven-year-old experience taught me that an overactive imagination worrying about what could go wrong had to be curtailed if life was to be fully lived. Once I began breathing again, my re-do Mediterranean swim went down as a victory (though I can't lie, I was still sure all kinds of sea creatures were hovering below me, just waiting...).

As I mentioned earlier, I had no idea what I was learning in the midst of these life experiences: moving to a new country, re-learning the meaning of words, creating new bonds and friendships, being different, trusting yourself to take on new challenges, and not allowing an overactive imagination to cast a shadow over what may be a great new experience.

However, looking back, these lessons—and many others—helped pave the way to accept the decision made by our children to also experience the adventures life has to offer. One such announcement was that our son, daughter-in-law, and six grandkids were moving from just down the street to accept a job... *in Ireland!*

My life experiences provided the peace to be OK with the decision, made by that same son, to travel in Europe with his family as digital nomads for five years. It may have been unconventional, filled with challenges, but what an amazing adventure! And it provided the impetus for us to visit them in some wonderful places and experience such fun times with our grandkids.

Life is the greatest teacher of all. All the lessons learned from these lived personal and family experiences left their mark on me, they informed who I am today, and how I view the world around me. They were also instrumental in inspiring a wonderful research focus when I moved from industry to academia. I wanted to dive into and learn everything I could about all things remote-work-related. This inspiration was foundational as I—and my hubby—laid out plans to live a mini version of the digital nomad lifestyle, in other words, working online while choosing where we want to live, just for a year.

One year... six locations? Four locations? That was still to be determined, and many details were yet to be ironed out. However, it did happen, and it was great! Many more stories have been added to our life lived.

CHAPTER 2

*"Travelling—it leaves you speechless,
then turns you into a storyteller."*

—Ibn Battuta

When I think of elements in life that have defined me, travel has got to be in the top five. But how do you take the lived experiences from visiting twenty-five plus countries over the course of sixty-one years, and combine them into one short chapter?

Imagine weekends heading to Annalong, the small fishing village in Ireland where my dad grew up. Fancy dress parades in the English gardens of a grand, old boarding house in the South of Ireland. Eating fish and chips on the pebble beaches of Portsmouth and Bournemouth, England, protecting the yumminess from hungry seagulls. As a young girl, I was enthralled as the Loch Ness Monster appeared through the foggy waters in the Scottish Highlands. After immigrating to Canada, even though our finances were tight, our family still managed to vacation in beachfront cabins that provided front-row seats to weather that lit up the sky, causing our hair to stand on end. We giggled at the sight we must have been, lying in bed with umbrellas protecting us from the effects of rain dripping through a holey roof. From storms that terrified us, to heat that had our virgin Irish skin running for cover, great memories were being created I'll never forget the road trips our family took to Disney World in Florida when four long days of mind-blowing boredom on unending highways were immediately forgotten when our eyes feasted on the magic that would create memories never to be erased.

It's even difficult to choose a few highlights... Every location—with its unique sights, sounds, smells, tastes, and fee— is worthy of more time and words than these pages allows. So, I'll take a different approach and consider some of the ways travel has impacted and informed my life.

The first lesson, *travel, like all of life, is most enjoyable when shared with others*. For example, several years ago, I presented at a leadership conference in Moncton, New Brunswick, then continued to Halifax, Nova Scotia on business. I had a free afternoon and decided to visit Peggy's Cove. It was early spring, so tourist season had not yet kicked in. I sat on the rocks looking out at the Atlantic Ocean, totally in awe of its power and awesomeness. But something was missing, I needed to share it with someone. Thank goodness for cell phones! For the next hour, I used texting and FaceTime to share the experience with my family, magnifying it a hundredfold. When visiting each of those twenty-five countries, every moment was shared with family or friends.

Second, *relationships are strengthened when experiences are shared*. Imagine climbing the 462 steps to walk around the outside of the Duomo in Florence, Italy, following a dander around the inside of the dome. The views, the architecture, the magnitude of the structure, the hundreds of people equally in awe of this wonder... who could resist reaching up and touching those amazing frescos? Apparently, everyone but me! Within seconds of *the touch*, an army of security guards came from all directions yelling, "*non toccare! non toccare! don't touch!*" I see with my fingers (a trait passed down to my youngest granddaughter, Abby, and grand-niece, Evelyn), how could I not touch? Needless to say, not only did I learn how much of a kinaesthetic learner I am, but my travelling friends have rehearsed that scene over and over, bringing us all to laughter as we relive the shared experience.

From the wonder of the Duomo to the heart-wrenching history behind the Ruin Bars found in the dilapidated Jewish ghettos in Budapest, such shared experiences can only deepen the bonds of relationships. On a trip to visit our kids in Ireland, Google Maps unexpectedly took us down Shankill Road in Belfast—not the best route! This route took us past murals painted on walls of buildings commemorating and—to my horror—celebrating the atrocities that took place during Ireland's Troubles. Tears immediately spilled from my eyes, and an instant panic attack set in. Once I was able to speak again, my shocked son and grandkids learned first-hand what life had been like as a young girl growing up in such turbulent times. Even as I write this, the memory of that day still brings me to tears. Our conversation that followed reached a depth only made possible by sharing that experience.

Third, *talking about travel is one of the best ways to build a connection between people*. I have the privilege of teaching culturally diverse classes at the Okanagan School of Business. Each semester brings a new group of international and domestic students, who often segregate themselves from one another. It's not because they don't like each other, it is simply a reflection of them not knowing or feeling comfortable with individuals from other countries and cultures. The domestic students that do not fall prey to this division are those who have experienced travelling to other parts of the globe; their worldview has been expanded and their sense of wonder has been fostered. What is even greater is when curiosity is birthed and the class as a whole begin learning from the many experiences shared by their travelled classmates.

I have taught many students from Europe (my favourite place to travel) and greatly enjoyed talking about visiting their home cities and countries. I remember one such conversation with a student from Berlin. I related how in June 2018, my son and I had travelled together in Europe for two weeks, conducting research on remote workers. Nathan, himself a remote worker and sojourner in Europe, had previously visited the amazing, historical city. While there, we toured the Berlin Cathedral on Museum Island, climbing two hundred steps to the Dome, ate bratwurst from street vendors, and visited two fantastic coffee shops: Five Elephant and The Barn (best peanut butter sandwich cookies ever!). However, the pleasures of the day were quickly overshadowed by a deep reverence as we walked through the Memorial to the Murdered Jews of Europe. What a sobering reminder of the horror lived by so many. That travel experience provided me with so many points of connection with my German students—as well as fodder for conversations with other students.

Four, *travel opens your mind to new ways of thinking, being, and doing*. During my first visit to Finland, I was struck by a prevailing attitude of "why not?", evidenced by these lovely people. The reason for my visit was to present at a global colloquium hosted by JAMK, University of Applied Science in Jyvaskyla. The focus of the conference was applied research, looking at the potential of academia collaborating with industry. Professors from many countries shared their research and learnings. In discussions, never once did I hear someone from Finland even hint at why something might not work. They listened with open minds and added to ideas rather than diminish those offered. This why-not attitude informed their daily lives. Why not go out for dinner at 11 p.m. in the middle of June while enjoying their *white nights*, a month when daylight lasted almost twenty-four hours a day? Why not find a peaceful spot in the middle of Esplanadi Park for a picnic accompanied by a glass of wine? Why not jump into the frigid Allas Sea Water Pool, when it is only two degrees Celsius out, in the middle of February?

From childhood through adulthood, travel adventures leave their mark. While in the midst of the journey, we may be unaware of how these marks, or influences, are being tattooed onto our psyche, our values, passions, future hopes, and life choices. Often, perhaps unintentionally, we impress these influences on our future life partners, children, and even friends. This certainly has been the case in my life. My husband of forty-five years was eager to embrace this tradition of yearly holidays in our marriage, and our children grew up expecting to have a holiday that involved family and oftentimes, friends. No matter how much, or how little, our budget would afford, we were able to welcome new adventures and experiences, creating a solid foundation towards embracing a healthy worldview of life. And, in case you are wondering, our two children and their families are building their own travel memories, some of which we've had the privilege of sharing with them.

Have our friends been similarly influenced? Yes! My husband and I are gleefully guilty of introducing two specific friends to the wide world of travel. For our twenty-fifth wedding anniversary, we decided to embark on a Mediterranean cruise. Of course, we shared this planned adventure with this couple, who shared it with two other couples (my husband and I had often travelled together with these good friends within North America). Before we knew it, all eight of us were totally immersed in planning "our" celebratory holiday. This was a new travel experience for the first couple—an experience they have since been repeated more times than I can count! To say they are addicted to such adventures would be an understatement.

But what if the privilege of travel is curtailed? I must confess, I have never for a moment considered what life would be like without the opportunity to travel when time and finances allowed.. I recently read an article forecasting what travel may look like post-COVID-19—not for a short period of time, but moving forward. The author revealed the many changes, such as fewer people on flights to allow for spacing, mandatory masks, frequent sanitising, janitors on all flights, gloves, flight attendants in protective gear, no in-seat movies, and longer processing times at the airport, to name a few. The author also suggested that some smaller airlines may need to close due to the rising costs of doing business. The bottom line? Fewer passengers and greater operating expenses equals increased costs, and passengers will be the ones to carry the burden.

How much more valuable will this make any opportunity to travel? Something I have so unconsciously taken for granted has now become a treasured experience. Perhaps where we travel and when we travel will be more intentional, more purposeful. As one reporter said, quick getaways will be replaced with more extended, planned-out travel. What would that mean for my travel year?

It's no wonder I strongly believe we should take advantage of every opportunity that comes along and embrace the many wonders and adventures life has to offer. How could I not have taken on an extended study leave that would afford me the opportunity to experience more of this amazing world we live in, learning from every encounter that comes along... and, even better, share some of it with family and friends? Saint Augustine said it so well: "The world is a book and those who do not travel read only one page."

CHAPTER 3

Expectancy is the atmosphere for miracles.
—Edwin Louis Cole

One year, twelve months, fifty-two weeks, 365 days. That's a long time. It represents a lot of missed time and experiences: time with family and friends, our chairs vacant for milestone events in the lives of our loved ones. Time missed sitting on the bench by the lake on warm summer evenings as we secretly sip wine from opaque water bottles, blinded by the bright ball of fire sinking down behind the distant hills. We would be missing out on the anticipation of the lilacs near our home bursting open, expelling their intoxicating fragrance, and the blossoming of wild roses. Missed joy, looking forward to the promise of spring as we huddle in a sheltered corner on the patio of our favourite coffee shop. Missing traditions, like my yearly pre-Christmas decoration-shopping date with my daughter, and the quiet moments spent sipping on eggnog as my husband and I finish decorating the tree for that much-loved time of the year.

Screeeech! (That's the noise of a needle being dragged over a record.) Let's back up here and refocus. We knew being away from home for one year would without a doubt come with a great sense of FOMO (fear of missing out). However, this was not a sad tale! This was my dream, my adventure, my idea. But a dream, an experience shared, is multiplied a hundredfold (at *least*) when shared. As you already know, my travel buddy, my co-conspirator, my dream-sharer, was my husband of forty-five years.

Let's back up to where this conversation started: Salou, Spain. It was February 2019. My husband and I were walking along the water's edge, the sand squishing between our toes as the warmth of the sun did its work making my freckles reproduce. I was feeling somewhat zombie-like following eight hours staring at the bedroom ceiling. One of *those* nights, on the heels of endless hours flying from Canada to Europe. However, it was not unproductive. Eight hours of uninterrupted think-time can give birth to surprising clarity.

Our beach walk soon found us enjoying the European practice of sipping wine and beer, eating olives and nuts, gazing out over the Mediterranean in the off-season, sleepy town of Salou, where our son and his family were spending six months of their travels.

"I wonder what the weather's like at home," Rob commented.

"Hmmm" was all I could mutter. "Who cares?"

"This is perfection!"

Then we fell into silence, each in our own thoughts, until the idea could no longer be contained.

"So," I said, "as I was staring at the ceiling all night rather than sleeping, I came up with an idea." I could hear Rob's unspoken *uh-oh*.

Taking a deep breath, I excitedly blurted out the plan I had concocted in the wee hours of the morning.

"For my extended study leave year, what do you think of spending it travelling in Europe, maybe living in four, even six different locations?" Inhale, then: "We would be able to embrace each culture and experience working fully remote. It would give me such great insight as to the practical side of what it truly means to not live in the same geographic location as either your team or organisation. We could rent out our condo for the year. You'll be retired. What do you think?"

A short, pregnant pause, and then…

"OK, sure." No drama, no "let's take some time to think it through," no "but what if…", just "sure!" No convincing needed. He was always open for a new adventure.

This was the first of many conversations with friends, family, and co-workers, all offering resounding affirmations, along with a few "better you than me!" However, the conversations that mattered most were those that took place with our kids and grandkids.

The first such a chat happened the very next day, with our son and his family—the ones already living a digital nomad lifestyle.

"That's amazing!" was Nathan's response. Crystal, our daughter-in-law, echoed the sentiment.

"Cool!" rang out a chorus of six excited voices ranging in age from five to fourteen. "Will you live with us for some of that time?"

"Are you kidding? Of course, we will… as long as you have room."

"You can have our room, Papa and Grandma." Generosity, personified.

The conversation proceeded to produce a flood of suggestions as to where we should spend that year; many of the ideas were based on memories of places Nathan and his family had lived over the past few years: Ireland, Portugal, France, Netherlands, Germany, Spain, Italy, and Finland. (You'll find the specific locations where our son and his family lived over a six-year period in the graphic above, created by our grandkids.)

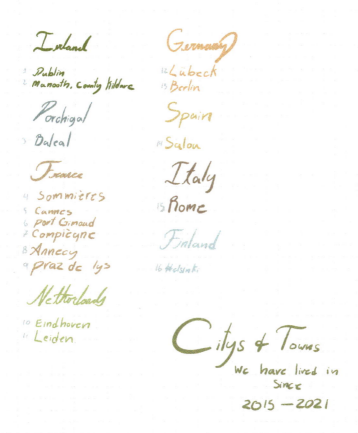

There wasn't an ounce of hesitation around our living away from Canada for an extended time —this kind of living had become the norm for our son and his family. Even though we had visited them in most of the places they lived, the realisation they might actually get to see us more often over the course of that year added to their exuberance.

However, the conversation took on a somewhat different nature with our newly-married daughter living close by in Kelowna.

"Oh, that's great," came the pensive response. "I've never gone a year without seeing you… I'm not sure I can do that!" Tears welling up.

"Shannon, there's no way we can go that long without seeing you, either… you'll come and visit us along the way." Our tears working in unison.

"Where?"

"Wherever you and Jordan would like to travel most."

While there was no doubt our daughter and son-in-law would fully support us, there wasn't the same shared joy at the announcement. I should have anticipated that. You see, even though our children were raised in the same home, by the same parents, with the same values, equally loved and encouraged to be who they are and follow their dreams and passions, they are unique individuals who approach life differently. Nathan loves an adventure and is always ready to go anywhere, anytime; Shannon is more measured and needs time to adjust to change. Given time, she is also ready for an adventure. We needed to give her time.

The other important dynamic had to do with the fact we would be moving closer to Nathan and his family while moving away from Shannon and hers. Understandable that our European kids would be more excited than those we were leaving back in Canada.

An important thing to keep in mind when we present ideas or plans to others is to remember we have had time to think, ponder, analyse, ideate, revise, and sit with these plans for an extended period of time. Rather than bursting forth in our exuberance with news of an exciting adventure, we need to afford others the same opportunity to think about, ponder, analyse, and sit with these ideas or plans—no matter how seemingly insignificant they may be. I should have taken this approach with Shannon. While she wasn't thrilled with the fact we would be gone for an extended period, we could at last freely discuss our plans and how we would keep connected… and of course, when and where they would come to visit us! That's where the conversation took on a more accepting quality. Yes, we might be away from Canada for a year, but not from our family for the full stretch of time—we were only ever a plane ticket away. We had instilled the importance and thrill of travel in our children, and we were now banking on that conviction to turn this adventure into a shared lived experience—one that included both of them.

While I was aware that our decision to pack up and leave the country for an extended period of time would impact those closest to us, I was perhaps not as cognisant of how much impact it would have on others. The decision we made called for much thought and consideration, and many reality checks. The most important people to us are family, closely followed by friends. I had no desire to say adieu to loved ones for a year of my life; they are my joy, my inspiration. And they would be part of this journey.

At that early time in our planning, a global pandemic such as COVID was something that lived in the minds of science fiction writers or doomsayers. That all changed in March 2020, a year after our plan hatched in Salou. Having already worked remotely for some time, I was confident in our ability to stay virtually connected with family and friends. However, before such a global event entered the picture, many people in our circle of friends were not as comfortable with technology. I knew we could stay connected, but forced isolation created the impetus for those wanting to stay connected with others to use tools such as Zoom in order to find a visual, virtual link to the outside world. Let's be honest: it's not as rich or fulfilling as being physically present, but it certainly goes a long way in nurturing already-established and valued relationships.

As I think back to 1970 when our family immigrated from Ireland to Canada. I can only imagine the pain experienced by our two sets of grandparents as the five of us climbed onto that plane to jet us away to the other side of the world. Neither my parents or grandparents had any idea when, or if, we would ever see each other again. As an almost twelve-year-old, my focus lay on the adventure ahead, not the relationships left behind. Making phone calls was very expensive at that time... no such thing as FaceTime or Zoom to stay connected and engaged with those loved ones left behind in our home country. I remember the tedium of writing letters on the special airmail letter paper, folding along the dotted lines, paying for an overseas stamp that cost fifteen cents per ounce, representing the international letter rate (the *really* thin, lightweight paper). Letter scribed and mailed, our grandparents would hopefully receive it in two to three weeks. By the time we received a reply, we couldn't even remember what questions we had asked—never mind what happenings we had reported!

If one needed to get an important message delivered, the faster choice was via telegram. Our family always had a house phone, but for those not quite as fortunate, a public phone was used to call the telegraph company and scribe the message. Because you paid for each word, the messages were intentionally brief. The original Twitter!

Fortunately, those days of challenging communications are long gone. For us, I knew that while we were physically apart from those precious friends and family, we would still be able to stay connected, virtually living life together. That combined with the hope and desire for those same folks coming to visit us, very quickly changed the conversation from that of sadness over separation, to joyous expectation, as they eagerly anticipated joining our adventure. The possibility of having them be a significant part of our lived experience, adding to the many memories we had already created by travelling together to far regions of the world, warmed my heart.

Our expectancy for this adventure was great, and it continued to grow the more we vicariously lived it, before it even began. Who knew that a decision conceived in the middle of a sleepless night in Spain would grow into an adventure to be planned and enjoyed by six adults and seven children, and, shared with friends both old and new?

CHAPTER 4

You'll never get anywhere if you go about what-iffing like that.
—Roald Dahl

"What if... ?" is the great crippler. Think about it: how many people use this question in a positive sense? What if I win the race? What if the sun shines on our wedding day? What if I don't get sick on this trip? What if I don't make a fool of myself? Rather, we worry about losing the race, having a special event rained out, getting seasick, or being humiliated over a poor performance.

These what-if questions can consume us to the point of paralysis. I remember standing on the second-highest diving board of the local outdoor, seawater-fed swimming pool in Bangor, Northern Ireland. Frozen (not just because of the Baltic temperatures), I rehearsed all the horrors that could mark the outcomes of a failed landing. Or—even worse—the humiliation of retreating to ground level. *It's now or never*, I remember thinking just before taking the step of no return. My nose was held tight by shaking fingers, it was the longest fall of my life. The positive what-ifs won. What if I make it? What if my friends are totally impressed with my bravery? What if the water is bathtub-warm by the time I land? (*Didn't happen.*) And it wasn't the last time I stepped off that platform.

In March 2020, most of us were living in isolation due to COVID-19. The what-ifs were very real. Our concerns around elderly parents, a pregnant daughter, children living in other parts of the world, family members with health issues, and friends losing their livelihoods were very real.

In fact, fast forward to mid-May, and I had just posted the following blog entry:

> *It's almost the end of the week. One more day. Actually, it's the Victoria Day weekend and I long for even two days to shut down and be totally offline. How quickly life has changed from truly enjoying connecting with folks virtually, to being so screen-weary that the thought of settling in with a real, hold-in-your-hands book is ripe with anticipation.*
>
> *Don't get me wrong, I love the times I get to visit and work with individuals across physical distance. I am truly blessed to participate in thought-provoking, encouraging, challenging, and mind-expanding conversations with amazing folks around the globe. But I miss going to a coffee shop for a visit with a good friend, or simply having a dedicated, productive time working while sipping on a rich americano created by one of my favourite baristas.*
>
> *It's the small things I miss. Happy hours on a patio catching up on the happenings of life around us, bike rides that end with a dark beer at a local brewery, hugging friends at will, holding a new-born baby without fear of endangering their fragile life, and sitting by the bedside of a dad who still remembers me. Planning weekend getaways to... anywhere!*

Still, I have much to be grateful for. I have a job I enjoy, I'm in good health, have a safe home in which to dwell with an amazing husband, I have a loving family who is committed to staying connected without compromising each other's health, am blessed with a great community of friends who make the extra effort to reach out and share life, I have amazing colleagues with whom to create and plan, am fortunate to live in a town/province/country where residents respect the need to band together to fight this crazy virus, and I have purpose.

But it's tough. I have deep empathy for those who must live life in compromising environments, not always of their own choosing. I struggle with isolation, even though my days are filled with virtual conversations, and I long for the days when we can confidently plan to meet up with loved ones who live in far-off lands. It will happen again, I know that. But for now, life is not what any of us expected—or even dreamed of.

It's… well, it's life! Let's pray for a brighter tomorrow.

A couple of days after I penned those words, those leaders we respect most began opening life up, very gradually. Still, the what-ifs grew. What if it was too early? What if people took the partial opening too far? What if the unspeakable happened and another, more serious wave hit? What if… ? There were no answers, only speculations.

Our doubts gave birth to more paralysing thoughts. It would be reasonable if the doubts we experienced throughout life were limited to such global pandemics, but they are not. As we considered leaving the life we enjoyed in British Columbia, trading it for a year travelling while working remotely, many what-ifs continued to bubble to the surface. What if one of us got sick?

What if we couldn't find suitable accommodations? What if we couldn't stay within our budget? What if we weren't able to rent our home out? What if we didn't see our daughter and son-in-law and new baby for a year? What if another pandemic hit? What if my dad passed away while we were gone? What if a family member or close friend had a crisis? What if I went through all the planning and the funding proposal was rejected? And—reality check—what if travel and work abroad were no longer an option due to whatever our new normal might be? It was crippling just thinking about all the potential challenges.

Those what-ifs were not insignificant. The small things in life do seem to have the greatest impact... what if I became obsessed with those small things when consumed with inevitable homesickness? Would I be able to move past the worry of potential challenges in order to witness glimpses of wonder as we set out on our adventure? Would I, like C. S. Lewis, remain open so as to be *surprised by joy*?[1]

And what if I *had* passed up such an opportunity? What experiences and adventures might I never have had, never have shared with my family and friends when they came to visit? Which lessons might I have lost out on? Which relationships might never have been built?

But what if my project *did* get approved, and all this planning became a reality? This kind of thinking made me start to feel giddy with possibility. Nothing about my situation had changed. I was no closer to having the trip planned or approved. However, my outlook and state of mind had changed—and my level of excitement increased to the point of bringing a big, dopy smile to my face while adding a few BPM to my heart rate.

What if we chose to face each day, each adventure, each

---

1 C.S. Lewis, *Surprised by Joy: The Shape of My Early Life*, (HarperOne; Reissue edition, 2017)

challenge with its positive potential in mind? What if we faced life with expectancy, like a child on Christmas morning, rather than channelling Winnie the Pooh's dear old friend Eeyore? What if our new normal brings opportunities and innovations that may never have emerged without the pain of a pandemic?

A remote year of travel would be influenced by how I chose to face both the joys and challenges presented. What if it truly turned out to be the greatest year ever? This became my focus.

CHAPTER 5

Curiosity creates connections.
—MICHELLE TILLIS LEDERMAN

I stood on the outside balcony of the beautiful lakefront hotel. The sun shone, the lake sparkled, the music volume was at just the right level for conversation, and every one of the 400 people in attendance was thoroughly enjoying themselves. Make that 399—I was not. My heart was racing, my palms were sweaty, and I wanted to bolt!

Just the day before, I and four other new business start-ups had agreed to go to the highest-attended annual networking event in Kelowna. You know, safety in numbers. None of us were comfortable selling ourselves to a crowd of strangers. So, we set a plan in place. We would pair up, approach the attendees, smile, have our new, shiny business cards ready to hand out and collect all the cards we could. We were prepared. What could possibly go wrong?

So, there I was, right on time, standing on the balcony like the Queen of England waiting to greet her subjects. That's when my cell vibrated with a notification of a text.

"I'm so sorry, but I can't make it tonight, something's come up."

"That's OK," I replied, "these things happen."

No problem, three of us can still work the plan. Just breathe, Roberta.

Then, another vibration.

"I hate to do this, but I just don't feel good. I need to bail tonight. You understand, don't you?"

Two down, two still standing. We got this! My breaths were almost coming in spasms. And then the unthinkable happened. You guessed it.

"My boyfriend just came into town for a surprise visit! I can't leave after he drove all this way. Sorry. I knew you'd understand."

I would understand? Are you kidding me?! I could have come up with a million valid reasons (OK, maybe two or three) for not making the event, but I didn't. I was there. I was alone. The air had been sucked out of my bubble!

Let me just insert here that I am truly an introvert. When I teach or present at a conference, you would never know it, but I am. If I'm representing something—or someone else—or if I have a task to do at a function, I'm OK. But put me in a situation with strangers and charge me with drawing attention to myself, and I'm not a happy camper. I'm in panic mode.

What happened next made me believe in angels. As my eyes scanned the crowd, they spotted a lady I had recently met. Our eyes met. She recognised me! And she was waving for me to come and join her! Thank you, God! When I reached the spot where she stood waiting, I quickly blurted out my dilemma, hardly stopping to breathe, and asked if I could hang out with her. I had only recently met this lady, so I'm sure my emotional eruption must have taken her aback. Her next words were music to my ears: "Of course, you can. Let me introduce you to some people and show you how it's done."

For the next two hours, I witnessed what I could only describe as "the networking dance." This lady moved fluidly from conversation to conversation, introducing me, asking questions of each person, smiling, inquiring about their lives, all the while holding onto a glass of wine, passing out business cards, and simply floating. I slowly released the breath I had been holding for so long. I was in awe!

My heart was no longer racing. I could shake someone's hand without fear of leaving a sweaty impression. I heard myself laughing and asking questions. I was actually having fun.

That was the moment I made a discovery,—had a lightbulb moment, worth every bit of anxiety I had ever experienced. Networking was not about telling people about me! It was about listening, paying attention to what others say—hearing their struggles, their joys, their pain—and, if appropriate, offering myself, my product, or my service to help meet their needs. That's it.

Being an introvert is actually a strength when in these situations. We don't need to be the centre of attention or the life of the party. Rather, we get to facilitate *others* being the life of the party.

As I travel to different countries, present at conferences, and meet new people, I still feel like the ocean undertow is threatening to suck me in. Having a co-worker (or hubby) with me is a lifeline, but not always possible. But when I remember to take my eyes off *me* and focus on others, I have been so gratified by meeting awesome people who are more than willing to tell me their stories. You see, networking doesn't just happen in huge crowds, but also between strangers standing on the train platform outside of Glasgow, waiting for a bus in Amsterdam, or having coffee in a local café in Florence. Networking is about connections (and I don't even like the term networking, anyway). Connections bring people together like a beautiful symphony produced when individual musicians join their skills and passions together to make music. Making new connections is worth the discomfort of sweaty palms, shortness of breath, and even fear of rejection.

CHAPTER 6

No one's life should be rooted in fear. We are born for wonder, for joy, for hope, for love, to marvel at the mystery of existence, to be ravished by the beauty of the world, to seek truth and meaning, to acquire wisdom, and by our treatment of others to brighten the corner where we are.

—DEAN R. KOONTZ

Choosing to see each day, each adventure, each challenge for its positive potential become our motto; a perspective both me and my husband (and family) were—and still are—choosing to live by. Much had happened. We now had a beautiful, adorable, healthy new granddaughter—Abigail Evelyn, named after the great-grandmother she would never learn to bake cookies with or learn to knit from, or even share a delicious ice cream cone with; a great-gramma who would have doted over her beyond measure. The joy she continues to bring to all of us is a blessing we certainly will never take for granted. Seeing our daughter and son-in-law transform into these amazing, loving parents wasn't a surprise, but nonetheless filled us with such pride and joy. Abigail's pictures, videos, and cuteness raised the *aww*-metre on a regular basis for her adoring cousins in Europe. Sadly, the picture also fed an inconsolable ache in the hearts of her Uncle and Auntie at not being able to cuddle her, whispering their unconditional love and commitment.

Then, there was the arrival of the unexpected. My husband began feeling unwell early in the year. After a myriad of tests and procedures, we received the news that his cancer of sixteen years past had resurfaced. Adding insult to injury, by the time he was able to get the diagnosis, his kidneys had been reduced to 8 percent functionality. In mid-August of 2020, he began kidney dialysis three times a week and chemotherapy every four. His final chemo treatment was in January. We hoped and prayed the treatment would once again arrest the cancer.... So far, so good!

Unfortunately, the news wasn't so good for his kidneys.

For six months every Tuesday, Thursday, and Saturday, at 5:30 p.m., you would find Rob bundling up in several layers of clothing, at the same time ensuring the layers would enable him to bare his chest for the dialysis tubes to attach to the port in his upper chest. For the next three to four hours, he would submit to the care of an amazing team of renal nurses and doctors as they did everything they could to keep him warm and comfortable, while the hemodialysis worked at cleaning the blood, getting rid of waste—basically, doing the work the kidneys were no longer able to do.

Eventually, what we feared most was voiced by the nephrologist: "The hope that once was clung to for kidney recovery has diminished. It doesn't look like they will recover. Unfortunately, you will need dialysis for the rest of your life." Such moments have the effect of putting life into slow motion. The words seeped into our conscious thought, then hit us with the force of Thor's hammer. Rob, always the eternal optimist, still hung onto a glimmer of hope that someday, his kidneys would fight back and become functional once more; however, as the days passed, that glimmer faded into oblivion.

In February Rob transitioned from hemodialysis to continuous ambulatory peritoneal dialysis (CAPD). Following three days of intense training for both of us, his dialysis treatment plan switched from three times a week at the hospital, to four times a day in the comfort of our home. Each exchange took forty-five to sixty minutes, making him feel like his IV pole was an added appendage. This transition wasn't without its challenges—finding the right solution strength, managing blood pressure and water intake, and ongoing changes in diet (difficult when one's desire for food is non-existent). It was a continuous process of hit-and-miss. Once Rob's body adjusted to the peritoneal dialysis, approximately two weeks after he switched, there would be another treatment transition—this time to automated peritoneal dialysis (APD), connected to a machine that would perform the dialysis while he slept. Thankfully, this would free him from the limiting four-times-a-day appointment for his drain-and-fill routine.

It was April 2020, and Rob had been on automated peritoneal dialysis for just over a week. I have to be honest: seeing the home dialysis machine on his bedside table took a bit of time to get used to. It stood (and still stands) as a monument reminding me that without the advances of modern medicine, without his nightly therapy with this new bedroom fixture, my husband would not survive more than two weeks. Those days, I found myself experiencing a certain kinship with Eyore, Winnie the Pooh's gloomy and sad donkey friend—though I still chose to believe that together, we would make it through.

But I quickly realised that in order to make it through, I needed to reach out for help. Burnout wasn't new to me. We all face challenges in life that require more help than a simple "put on your big girl panties" to make it through. These over-the-top challenges can blindside you. They have done that to me; the premature death of a child, a mom passing away in her mid-sixties with Alzheimer's, followed by a dad's final years of life being stolen by pre-senile dementia. With each overwhelming adversity, I fought, until I came to the end of myself and knew I had to reach out for help.

I knew I couldn't fight it alone. A visit to the emergency room during those dark days as we were adjusting to life with Rob's renal failure, served as a wake-up call that if I was to enjoy, relish in, embrace, and share my life, I needed to make some changes.

We all deal with challenges differently. Watching what my husband was going through I felt guilty complaining about not being able to sleep. There were some mornings I needed something to get me started. Coffee, even a little bit, would do. Even though I knew it was something my system could not tolerate, there were many days I simply needed a caffeine hit, even if it was one scoop of caffeine coffee mixed with my three scoops of decaf. Some days, that percentage grew to a full-on cup of regular coffee to give me the pick-up I needed to face the day after yet another sleepless night. Caffeine became my drug of choice, When explaining my reaction to the emergency room doctor: the rapid heart rate and palpitations, the high anxiety, the light-headedness, I received no sympathy—instead, "What were you thinking?" Point taken; lesson learned. It's been over two years since I've had a cup. But I sure do miss it! Thanks to support from doctors and friends, most days, I have also learned to deal with anxiety without medication... but sometimes, I still get blindsided and feel no shame in using an anti-anxiety pill to bring back homeostasis, allowing me to get on top of life again. We both know that life will never go back to what it was before my husband's diagnosis, that's our reality, but we get to choose if we will let that define us. We both need to keep asking ourselves what would happen if we chose to see each day, each adventure, each challenge, for its positive potential.

So, you see, sometimes, the what-ifs *do* become a reality, the pain of those life events we never want to realise. But sometimes, those much hoped-for what-ifs blossom into life, the dreams we loosely held on to actually come true.

At the end of November 2020, in the midst of struggling through life's unexpected twists and turns, I received an email from our college president that brought me such joy and excitement, I was stopped in my tracks!

> *Dear Roberta, regarding your proposal for an extended study leave, I am pleased to advise that your proposal has been approved as follows:*
>
> *August 1, 2021 to July 31, 2022, in Europe, for the purpose of conducting research that will examine what it takes to lead successfully in a new, uncharted working context that has been coined a "new normal."*

Looking back to that day, it still gives me shivers to realise we made the adventure happen in spite of the obstacles before us. What if, indeed!

CHAPTER 7

*The world is so much larger than I thought.
I thought we went along paths, but it seems there are no paths.
The going itself is the path*
—C. S. Lewis, *Perelandra*

I'm a planner—always have been, and always will be. I have a need to look forward, to think ahead, to anticipate possibilities. Once I start planning, it's difficult to shut my mind off. The prospect of a full year dedicated to researching and learning about leadership in complex, hybrid, and work-from-anywhere teams had my mind running at full speed. *And doing all that while living in another part of the world!* Planning is part of the adventure. I've been responsible—by myself or as part of a team—for planning everything from small family events to weddings, to special-occasion parties, to vacations, to conferences hosting a thousand or more attendees. I love it! But planning for an extended time away conducting research while working through a severe medical issue with my travel partner would be the planning event of my life. I know it sounds a little dramatic, but believe me, it was the truth!

During this mind flurry, a persuasive part of me—a small but unrelenting voice—constantly urged me to slow down and lean into my areas of strength, enabling me to lay a solid foundation for an amazing year.

Very early in my planning, this inner voice prompted me to consider my strengths and blind spots. I'm passionate about the need for leaders to know themselves, and in so doing, lead themselves before stepping up to lead others. I decided that time would be well spent reviewing the results of my StrengthFinder assessment, an amazing tool created by Gallup. Let me share some of my report's insights (in no order of relevance):

- It's very likely you might be eager to get started on a project once you realise what can be accomplished in the coming weeks, months, or years.
- Your mind allows you to venture beyond the commonplace, the familiar, or the obvious.
- You can make things happen by turning thoughts into action.
- You refuse to be stifled by traditions or trapped by routines.
- You bristle when someone says, "We can't change that. We've always done it this way."
- You enjoy looking at the world from different perspectives and are always searching for connections.
- You feel confident in your ability to take risks and manage your own life.
- You have an inner compass that gives you certainty in your decisions.
- You are intrigued by the unique qualities of each person.
- You can figure out how different people can work together productively.

- You love to learn, and you intuitively know how you learn best.

- Your natural ability to pick up and absorb information quickly and to challenge yourself to continually learn more keeps you on the cutting edge.

And the blind spots I needed to watch out for? Here are some that hit the *ouch*-button for me:

- Because you typically do not trust others implicitly and people have to earn your trust over time, some may think you are hard to get to know.

- When working with others, sometimes, people may misinterpret your strong strategic talents as criticism.

- Sometimes, you might charge ahead and act without a solid plan B.

- Because you speak with authority, you might be used to getting the final word.

- Before you commit to something, make sure you have the time and resources you need to do it right.

- You love the process of learning so much that the outcome might not matter to you. Be careful not to let the process of knowledge acquisition get in the way of your results and productivity.

So, with all that in mind, I was compelled to slow down, take a breath, create a plan, and follow it! The criteria of what I needed to accomplish on this study leave was laid out, thanks to the demand for a thought-out proposal required by the college. The plan I created addressed everything to be arranged before we hit *go* on the first of August 2021, and it identified all the expected learning outcomes from the research. The plan was about laying the foundation and had to be determined before jumping into my many research activities in various locations, before meeting amazing people, and before embracing new experiences. Time and focus first had to be given to the planning... it had to take front seat in my mind.

Our original plan for this extended study leave involved living and travelling in Europe for a full year, spending time in six countries, taking advantage of cheap flights within the continent, and armed with only carry-on luggage. Simple, straightforward, and flexible. Then, the unexpected happened... a global pandemic and our own personal health challenges.

But, as I said, I'm a planner. So, I came up with a new plan. Eight months, two countries, and a rental car to get us from place to place. Our simple practice of only using one carry-on piece of luggage each had to change. The new practice included two carry-ons filled with dialysis solution and medical supplies—*and* one large, hard-cover case housing a dialysis machine (not-so-affectionately referred to as *the beast*). And of course, two larger checked suitcases to carry our clothes and additional medical supplies. The good news? It was totally doable!

I do find humour in how our lives keep transitioning. Our first major European vacation was in 2008. My husband and I, along with three other close friend-couples, boarded a flight from Vancouver, BC that would transport us to beautiful Florence, Italy. From there, we went on to Cinque Terre, then to Venice, where we boarded a cruise ship and spent the next twelve days exploring eight spectacular ports in Greece, Italy, and Spain. Imagine, if you will, eight adults, loaded down with luggage, getting on and off planes, trains, buses, ferries, and taxis, armed only with a knowledge of the English language and an immense sense of adventure.

I'm sure we provided great entertainment to myriad other travellers as they watched the group of us climbing up and down many steps, traversing from one train platform to the next... eight adults, eight good-sized suitcases, eight carry-on bags, eight knapsacks, and two smaller carry-on cases carrying medical supplies. I must take time to applaud one member of our party, a dear friend. She has a medical condition that requires her to bring solution with her no matter where she goes, to rehydrate through a port in her upper chest. Talk about not letting medical issues prevent you from adventure! Little did we know, those many expeditions with friends would provide us the encouragement and confidence to move forward with our European adventure.

But the humour doesn't stop there. If you have spent any time in Europe, you'll know that elevators are not a common mode of transporting people and their luggage to their accommodations—at least not the Airbnb-type places we frequented. I remember getting to our first reservation in Florence and being faced with four flights of stairs. Some of us moaned, some used expletives, others simply laughed. Then, up we climbed. Perhaps the craziest climb happened in Cinque Terre. After a hundred stairs, our travel mates reached their rooms. Not my husband and me. As we stood facing a wrought-iron spiral staircase of a hundred more steps, we started laughing.... But up we climbed, luggage and all. As is often the case after a great deal of effort, we were rewarded with a balcony room presenting a view of the Mediterranean that was nothing short of breath-taking. The climb was well worth it. Little did I know it was a foreshadowing for the three flights of stairs we would climb, luggage and medical supplies in tow, up to our flat in Valencia!

And so, for our new adventure, the climb would be well worth it. Together, Rob and I were about to embark on the adventure of a lifetime—unexpected flights of stairs to climb, multiple solution boxes to haul around, machines blowing up, many medical supplies to pack, and a great deal of lab work, were all part of the adventure to come. Life doesn't stop in your sixties, nor does a life-threatening illness have to chain you down.

So, what is involved in all this planning? Let me start with the basics.

1. Budget (the old 'money in - money out' equation)
2. Travel dates
3. Figuring out an itinerary... where we would actually go.
4. Potential flights and their costs (economy simply wasn't an option)
5. Accommodations while travelling (thank God for Airbnb!)
6. Transportation from place to place (Europcar did well for us)
7. Renting out our home while we travel (a big thanks to personal connections)
8. Travel insurance (no problem for me—I was covered under my medical plan. Rob, not so much.)
9. Travel Visas (I had a European passport for many years due to my Irish origins, so I was good to go. My hubby still needed one. Or so we thought... more on that later.)

Planning beyond the basics involved more....

1. Travel insurance for pre-existing conditions for extended travel (no one wanted to touch a dialysis client with a ten-foot pole except BCAA. All for the bargain price of $16,000. While others used unspent COVID money on house renovations, we were saving for travel insurance!)
2. Learning that the dialysis machine originally prescribed was not supported in Europe... then finding one that was.

3. Communication with airlines to confirm they would allow needles and liquid medical supplies and medicine on board—which also greatly exceed carry-on weight allowances—and attaining special valet check-in for a dialysis machine.

4. Choosing accommodations that had sufficient room for a month's worth of dialysis solution (forty-plus 12x13x14" boxes), which were also on the ground floor or with an elevator (though big surprises awaited us in Valencia).

5. Confirming that the locations we choose were places the medical supply company would deliver dialysis solution.

6. Contacting hospitals in each location to confirm we could access their services in case of a nephrology emergency—and for lab work.

The months of planning before we left were exhausting, to say the least. They were fraught with misinformation, questions with no answers, countless emails to the Portuguese consulate (the country we were to spend the first months of our sojourn), and communications with medical facilities in Spain where English was simply not spoken; very quickly, we realised that what we were doing was not "normal." We were pioneers in taking on such an overseas travel adventure, and while many wanted to help, there was just no information available to help us accomplish what was needed. So, we forged ahead, committed to making things work, and faced each challenge as it presented itself.

There are advantages to being a stubborn, tenacious Irish woman who won't back down from a challenge. That, and knowing we are blessed beyond measure with a group of amazing supportive friends. Some of us have known each other for around thirty-five years at the time I'm writing this… that's a long time! We have lived life together through the good times and the bad. Through grief, pain, and sorrow. Through celebrations, joys, and laughter. We have seen each other at our worst and at our best. These friends are truly gifts from God, gifts we will never take for granted. And they were right there to provide the encouragement and support to help us prepare for this new adventure.

Another part of planning and preparation was figuring out the logistics of travelling with a serious medical condition. Again, we came up with a plan to help prepare us for the unknown. We would take baby steps:

1. Local travel

2. In-province travel

3. Cross-Canada travel, and then

4. International travel.

When you are faced with such medical issues, the easiest thing is to pack away your luggage, put passports back in the safety deposit box, and explore the world through books—or by listening to others' adventures. I get that. But that's not what my husband or I wanted. However, we knew the way we had done things in the past wouldn't necessarily work for moving forward. We needed to relearn how to travel. This called for baby steps before we took the big leap across the mighty ocean.

In the early days of my husband's diagnosis, his medical team strongly suggested he create a "go-bag." Being a lover of espionage-type TV shows, movies, and books, I certainly understood the concept of a go-bag. It's all about being prepared for the next world crisis—or in our case, for whatever eventuality would prevent Rob from getting home to his dialysis machine at the end of the day. This meant four bags of dialysis solution and all the medical supplies necessary to create a sterilised environment and administer his dialysis. Check and check!

First baby travel step? A day trip to Salmon Arm, BC involving a beautiful 110-kilometre drive from our home, where we could enjoy a coffee stop along the way, a peaceful walk by the stunning Shuswap Lake, and a wander through some locally-owned shops. And, not to be missed, picnic lunch from the Shuswap Pie Company, where they serve up the most delicious savoury and sweet pies imaginable. So, with our go-bag ready, we were off. All in all, it was a successful first step... apart from the wind and rain that greatly curtailed our lake walk, having us inhale our pies for fear of getting drenched. We were ready to up the game.

Second baby travel step. A few of our friends decided that we needed a getaway... a chance to step away from routine and enjoy each other and the spectacular area in which we lived. For Rob's birthday, they gifted us with an overnight stay, including dinner and breakfast, at the charming Hester Creek Winery, about an hour-and-forty-five-minute drive from our home.

The most important things in life are not things
But rather, a series of moments of love, of relationships of memories
and experiences.

It starts with family and friends who are always there for you.
Their influence and support shape your character.
It's having that perfect person to do life with
...holding hands, walking on a sandy beach.
Nurturing a son and daughter—foundation of family.
The blessing of seven grandchildren... precious moments with
their Papa.

It is having friends who build into you...
Who hold you to account, who love to laugh and share,
And enjoy each and every adventure.
Who walk beside you with encouragement and support.

*It is incredible memories and experiences
Of children's first holidays and travel… your first motorcycle,
Quiet conversations over coffee… taking in the wonder of "littles"…
the grandeur of "bigs."*

*The intention of our gift
is to help create another special memory for you and Roberta.*

We love you.

(This letter, penned by Mrs. C, accompanied the gift)

See why our friends are truly a blessing to us?

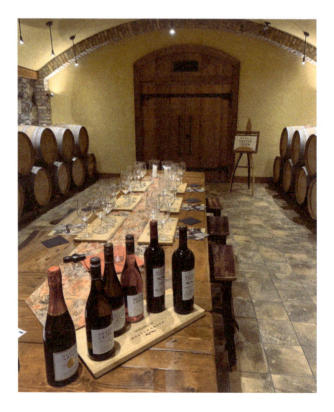

Hester Creek Winery

This adventure required more than a go-bag. Overnight meant we needed not only to pack dialysis solution and supplies, but also to haul the dialysis machine (the beast) with us, so Rob could plug in and do a full night's exchange. We could do it! Rob made a list of everything he needed, together we packed it all, and I lugged it to the car. Being on peritoneal dialysis meant that my hubby can't lift anything over twenty-five pounds. You can imagine how difficult it was for him to relinquish the task of heavy lifting to me… one adjustment among many. But off we went, and celebrated another victory as our second baby travel step was accomplished.

Third step (not quite so baby anymore): extended time away from home. The next trip had us packing up enough dialysis solution and supplies for a week. Our little Honda HRV was acting more like a truck as we made the drive to Vancouver, where we embarked on a ferry to make the crossing to Vancouver Island. We were so excited to get away to a place we so love to visit! Our confidence was mounting as we checked into an Airbnb, set up Rob's supplies and machine, and set out to explore beautiful Victoria, the capital of our province. We walked a lot (albeit much slower than we normally would), enjoyed sitting by the ocean, ate at a few of our favourite restaurants, and even drove up the island to visit a close friend of Rob's (bringing along the go-bag, of course!). We were learning that with a few adjustments, our travel adventures could still happen. As our friends expressed, it was time to create new travel memories—and that's exactly what we did.

But there's more… the fourth step, the biggest yet! Flying. Going to Europe involved getting on a plane, and with more than just our carry-ons, as we were accustomed to. With just over two months until we were scheduled to get on the plane in Vancouver to travel to Lisbon, it was time for the dress rehearsal. Thanks to a generous retirement gift from his boss and some travel credits (thanks to COVID), we were able to fly to Ontario without a great deal of expense. This was perfect, because my brother and his family lived there, so we had the assurance of knowing our accommodations would be more than adequate. Travelling by plane also meant greatly increased pre-travel communication with the airlines to make sure they would accommodate the dialysis machine without it being checked as well as allow a few bags of solution in our carry-on luggage (well over the maximum weight allowed). Assurances granted by the medical folks at the airlines, we were good to go. Apart from extra searching going through security, the letters provided by Rob's medical team paved the way for clearance to be quickly granted.

As I'm sure you've already realized, there was no way we were able to transport any more dialysis solution on the plane than two carry-on suitcases would hold. Baxter, the supplier of all things dialysis, stepped up. They delivered all the necessary supplies directly to my brother's home several days before we arrived. Honestly, we are so incredibly fortunate to have the kidney dialysis support we do across Canada… and, as we would soon learn, worldwide.

Our practising was complete: several day trips, two overnight trips, one in-province week-long trip, one four-thousand-plus-kilometre flight across Canada, and multiple lessons learned, we were as ready as we would ever be.

While this was going on, August arrived. It was time to focus on the actual research.

CHAPTER 8

Bizarre travel plans are dancing lessons from God.
—KURT VONNEGUT

Thirty-six thousand feet in the air, enroute to Portugal… I could hardly believe what had once been a dream had finally become a reality. Just a year ago, my proposal for extended study leave had been approved, and our plans for the year had begun to take shape. There had been many adaptations and workarounds, but we had done it; our eight-month adventure in Europe had officially begun.

The weight of how many hurdles we had had to overcome finally dissipated. Our Covid vaccinations had been administered at a local medical clinic, and clear results from pre-travel screening had arrived within the designated timeframe. *Phew*! Accommodations for our European adventure were all lined up, rental cars confirmed. There was nothing else to do.

I turned to Rob and said, "We did it! We are finally on our way!'

As I sipped on my welcome-aboard drink (we treated ourselves, basking in the luxury of business class), I took time to look back on the often-rocky path that had gotten us here.

The original plan had been to be in Europe for twelve months, to visit at least five countries, and to basically live life as digital nomads. You know the saying... *the best-laid plans*.... While the goal had remained the same, the plan had changed. The combination of the pandemic and my husband's kidney failure greatly tested our resolve to step out on this journey. But there we were, on the plane headed for Europe. For the next eight months, we would split our time between Portugal and Spain.

I had gained a whole new appreciation for people who put forth the effort to travel and live abroad for an extended time. We watched our son and his family pack up their six children and make the move to my home country of Ireland, the reverse of my parents' adventure when I had been a young teenager. I thought I had a reasonable understanding of the process. I was wrong.

Born in Ireland, living in Canada, I have both an EU and Canadian passport... very handy. In early spring, it was brought to our attention that my husband needed to have a visa to travel to Europe because of the length of our stay. So, we started the application process. Do you know how difficult—how frustrating—it is to find information on a website from a country that's not your own? Worse, that does not share the same language? After many emails and phone calls, a lovely person at the Portuguese consulate finally looked at the site and admitted, "Oh, yes! That is rather confusing, isn't it?"

You see, there wasn't an option for our situation. I wasn't going to Europe for a job, my husband was retired, we weren't travelling for medical reasons, I was not providing training and development, we weren't going to volunteer, I wasn't going to further my education. Without making this selection, you don't get access to the portal where the required documents, such as passports, can be uploaded and an visa application interview appointment made. So, I had to choose something, and they would fix it later. To make a really long story short, after a five-hour drive to Vancouver to visit the consulate—followed by more conversations—it turned out my husband didn't need the visa we were seeking. Instead, he had to go through a totally different process—once in Europe. We laugh about it now, but at the time this added even more stress to an already trying process.

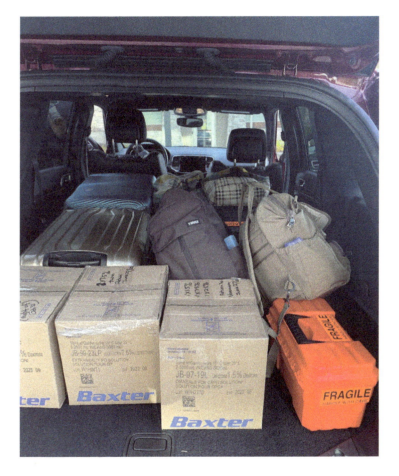

COVID also presented many potential barriers for travel, but we overcome them all. I never realised how many people you could call to try to find out the proper processes, tests, timing, and locations—without finding anyone who would give a definitive answer. Again, easy to laugh at now... but I can assure you, my Irish came out full force at times.

We learned that travelling with certain medical equipment was not common, so we began researching, asking questions, reading, seeking input, and making phone calls. Eventually, we learned that producing the proper papers provided by medical professionals, would allow us to proceed through airport security without too much scrutiny, So, with a dialysis cycler and transformer compatible with EU voltage, extra solution just in case, (all of which had to travel with us on the plane, not underneath in the baggage compartment), and more suitcases than we had ever travelled with, we were packed and ready to drive to Vancouver to catch a flight the following day for Lisbon via Toronto.

Without the help and support of an amazing family, great friends, a fantastic medical team, and the opportunity to take time away from teaching at Okanagan College School of Business to engage in research, we would not have found ourselves thirty-six thousand feet in the air, filled with excitement for what our adventure would hold.

Thankfully, our flights and connection in Toronto all went off without a hitch, and the next day, we arrived in Lisbon. We did—but not our luggage!

CHAPTER 9

Some things are so unexpected that no one is prepared for them.
—Leo Rosten

My appreciation and respect for people who choose to pack up and move to another country for a time continued to grow. After arriving in Lisbon, my research—and our adventure—continued. But to say our first week had some hurdles would be an understatement. We faced so many challenges, it was hard to believe we had only just arrived! As we look back on it, we aren't quite at the laughing point, though we have progressed to a head shake and slight groan. The memory still haunts me.

All our checked luggage had left Vancouver with us, but had decided to remain where we'd had our first layover—Toronto. You can imagine the frustration and anxiety we experienced when we discovered, two hours after we had arrived, that our luggage had not made it. Fortunately, the dialysis machine travelled with us via valet service… we actually brought it right to the door of the plane, so we knew it would arrive when we did. By this time, my husband desperately needed to get settled and hooked up for a dialysis treatment.

Beyond exhausted, we were grateful to our son for arranging

a valet taxi service to pick us up from the airport and deliver us to our Lisbon home. However, we didn't have a contact number to let the driver know what was going on. So, our son, who was in Finland, acted as the liaison, letting the driver him know the situation. Three hours later, we were finally in the van, heading through the narrow, winding, hilly, cobbled streets of Old Town Lisbon.

Once we had been delivered, my husband handed a card to the driver, with the intent to include a healthy tip. To our horror, his machine wasn't working, and we had no cash! We were amazed when the classy gent simply said, "Don't worry about it, we'll figure it out," and drove away! (It took a few weeks to finally figure out how we could pay him... which we were more than happy to do.) Quite the welcome to Portugal.

It took five days for our luggage to catch up with us, making it necessary for us to purchase some fill-in-the-gap clothing. Given the possibility our luggage might never arrive, we had to fill out a claims form outlining every single item in the suitcases—including the colour, size, brand, year purchased, and cost. Not an easy thing to do when working through jetlag. This luggage delay also meant we had to find supplements to purchase for my husband that had the same nutritional value as those in Canada. Fortunately, he had taken pictures to show the pharmacist.

Having to launder our travel clothes to alternate with our newly-purchased outfits was challenging when they took more than twenty-four hours to hang-dry. I took a picture of the outfit I pieced together from what had dried, and what had just been purchased and sent it to my girlfriends... no way you would have found me walking around Kelowna looking like that! We did get a good laugh from it (very welcome).

Then there's the transformer incident. This piece of equipment was necessary to operate my husband's Canadian dialysis machine in Europe. After using it for only two nights, it literally blew up. Thankfully a replacement dialysis machine was delivered by Baxter—one that did not require a transformer. However, *it* wasn't working. The next day, another replacement came. Fortunately, we were lucky the third time! We had taken our go-bag on the plane with us for this very reason. Once again, we were thankful for the wisdom of Rob's medical team.

While the location of our Lisbon home was great, we soon realised the power fuses would blow if too many appliances were running at the same time—so no coffee maker, toaster, kettle, anything extra, until Rob had finished dialysis. Sadly, with little natural light, our Airbnb felt rather cave-like. We also learned that the radiator didn't work, so we often found ourselves bundling up in sweaters.

We knew that once in Europe, we would need to order some products from Amazon. Interesting fact: you can't order from Canada while in Europe, nor can you order from Amazon in Portugal. However, you can order from Amazon in Spain, which would then ship to Portugal. Confusing, I know. And yes, the order needed to be completed in Spanish. Being a monolingual, this was a challenge. I was fairly sure I had ordered the right things, but until the products arrived at the end of the following week, all I could do was hope for the best. Good news… it was a successful order!

That was the glass half-empty story… now, the glass half-full perspective. The driver our son arranged was amazing. He waited for us at the airport and didn't even charge us for the extra wait time. We were so impressed. Our clothes did arrive, eventually, delivered right to our door with an apology. No need for a replacement wardrobe. And the pharmacists in Lisbon were great, helping us choose the best products, closest to what my husband used at home. Full marks for them!

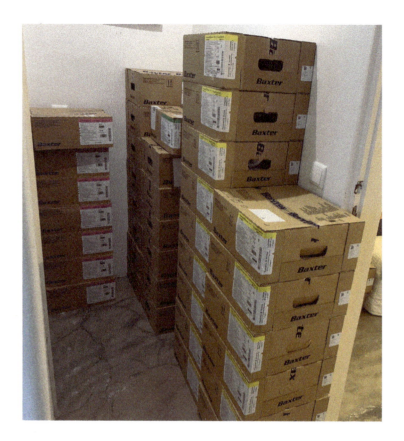

A month's supply of dialysis solution

Baxter, our supplier for all things dialysis, went above and beyond. Truly a lifeline. If you want to study what great customer service looks like across borders, look no further.

We learned to be more intentional in our use of electricity (limit it or lose it!). In the evenings, we would sit with a blanket around us and watch Netflix (no English channels were available on TV) until it was finally time to climb into a cozy bed. Truly a lovely memory of togetherness.

Because of the lack of natural light in our place, we spent a great deal of time outdoors, exploring Lisbon and finding third spaces to soak in the vitamin D while getting reading and research done. Through all of these bumps, our hostess was over-the-top amazing! She deserves twice as many hospitality stars as Airbnb allows.

Google Translate became my constant companion. We had planned on learning some Portuguese and Spanish before leaving Canada, but time got away from us. Again, we were greatly impressed with the graciousness of the Portuguese people—they were so hospitable in speaking English (even apologising for not speaking fluently enough!). The most Portuguese we could manage was *obrigada*, a word we used more times in a week than imaginable.

Lisbon is an incredible city. Every day, we set out in a different direction to see what we could find—and loved the surprises around each corner. Our flat was close to São Jorge Castle, in the Alfama Barrio, much higher in elevation than the main streets of Lisbon. As a result, every direction we went called for walking up and down steep streets. Lisbon certainly is the city of seven hills!

As we experienced the unexpected that first week, I was reminded of the research my son and I had published in 2019 focused on competencies for remote workers' success. Those competencies, we discovered, go well beyond work contexts. The freedom to work and live anywhere is a gift, but it also comes with the responsibility—personal and professional—to make things work. It's not easy to pack up and pursue such an adventure.

We thought through all the possible scenarios of what might happen, and we were confident we had contingency plans in place. We still were not fully prepared. When you pack up and leave, you are not only leaving your home, with all its conveniences, but you are also leaving your support network—familial, social, and medical. Sure, you can reach out via text, email, or phone if necessary (after figuring out where to purchase an EU SIM card and changing your messaging platforms to a new number), but with an eight-hour time difference, they might be fast asleep when you are in the middle of turmoil. Even though our son and family living in Europe, they were still a day's drive away. My husband and I had travelled to Europe several times, but this trip was not a vacation. I was born in Europe, but I had left as a young teen. What we experienced on this trip was all so different from vacation travel.

Did we regret the decision? Not for a moment! Would we recommend it to others? Without a doubt! Was it as easy as we anticipated? Not the first week. But there was so much more adventure to come.

During our time in Lisbon (more correctly, Lisboa), we lived in the Old Town and felt like we were part of the community. We loved speaking with the local business owners and storekeepers—mostly of small family operations. Their English was poor, our Portuguese non-existent, but still we were able to learn some of their stories. Most people walking around were tourists, but after a short time, we seemed to transition out of being tourists. At that time, we hadn't come up with a suitable description of what we were, though. We didn't really get to know anyone, but we soon recognised the residents as they were going to and from work. A favourite pastime—especially for my husband—was sitting in coffee shops in the historic area, taking in the sights and sounds. On our second evening, a local restaurant owner welcomed us to Lisbon with their local Ginjinha, a cherry liquor that was delicious. It felt good at the end of each day to climb the hills back to Old Town, return to our part of Lisboa, and enjoy a drink close by before returning to our flat.

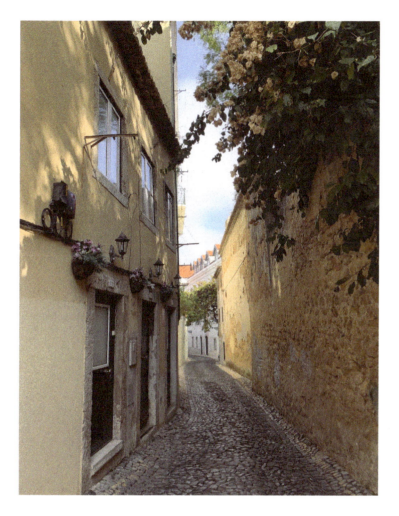

Santa Maria Maior

A short five-minute walk uphill was Sao Jorge Castle. On the corner, just before the castle, was a small wine and coffee bar that offered a delicious apple strudel served with their wonderful in-house ice cream. Their wine, like most in Portugal, was delicious and inexpensive. This quickly became Rob's favourite location to sit with a cup of coffee or glass of wine and watch people while I got work done. We soon got into a routine of working and exploring, thoroughly appreciating the beauty around us. I did not skip indulging in my daily *pastel de nata*. For those not familiar, it's a Portuguese egg custard tart pastry with a sprinkling of cinnamon on top that I quickly came to appreciate,—made, sold, and enjoyed all over Portugal.

We loved setting out to explore, and were thrilled when we would turn a corner to find ourselves in a place we actually recognised. One such exploration brought us to the sixteenth-century monastery of São Vicente. To say it was a step back in history doesn't even come close to what we experienced. The cloisters presented mosaics, paintings, statues, and beautiful azulejos. These blue ceramic tiles are one of the most unique art forms in Portugal. Venturing up a steep staircase, we were rewarded with the most spectacular view of Lisbon.

While we no longer felt like tourists, we would still put on our tourist hats to visit attractions like the oceanarium, art museums, and the LxFactory. This co-operative working venue, located right on the banks of the Tagus, is filled with unique store, cafes, restaurants, and galleries. Not long ago the area was just an abandoned factory yard. The LxFactory already held special memories for Rob and me—it was the first place our son and his family had taken us when I had arrived to join my husband in Lisbon on a previous trip. Each of these amazing places greatly contributed to our appreciation of the city.

Fado provided a deeper glimpse into the human history of the area. The soulful Portuguese folk music was filled with such passion. We were privileged to listen to a talented woman accompanied by two musicians at a restaurant just a five-minute walk away from our flat, who drew us in with their musical story of culture and tradition. Amazing, since we didn't understand a word they sang! The meal before the performance was also delicious and bountiful. We left with full stomachs and full hearts.

Lisbon was our first sojourn, but each place we stayed on our adventure became our home. And as most will recognise, certain challenges present themselves when transitioning to a new home. Here are some of the ones we found ourselves facing with each transition.

- Getting oriented to a new environment
- Finding a grocery store within walking distance
- Setting up a new home, including finding what necessities you need to purchase, finding out Internet access passwords
- Getting our cell phones set up in different countries
- Finding locations other than home to do my research in
- Learning to drive on unfamiliar (and sometimes very narrow!) roads
- Familiarising ourselves with local transportation
- Figuring out how to pay for various transportation modes
- Locating International Clinics
- Locating hospitals and finding the ones most likely to have English-speaking staff and nephrologists on staff
- Avoiding the temptation to live like a short-term tourist (budget matters!)

We were no longer tourists, yet we needed to avoid the temptation to live like a short-term tourist (budget matters!). In searching for a way to describe what we were, if not tourists, I came across this description of *sojourners* in a travel blog called Sojourner Tours.

"Several principles distinguish sojourners. The most obvious is that they organise their trips around a single location, or base, from which they can take day trips. Their objective is to immerse themselves in a new culture as much as possible by interacting with local people, eating regional specialties, and learning about the community's customs and beliefs.

They are open to new experiences and enjoy adapting a bit. In the end, they judge the success of their trips not just by the number of famous sites they photograph but *also by how deeply their experiences affect and enhance the way they live once they return home.*[2]"

This was something we could relate to…we were Sojourners.

---

2 "Are You A Sojourner?" Sojourner Tours, accessed April 10, 2023, http://www.sojournertours.com/organized-small-group-tour-participant-characteristics.

CHAPTER 10

It was the best of times; it was the worst of times....
—Charles Dickens, *A Tale of Two Cities*

One of my desires for this memoir is to present an honest, transparent glimpse into our time in Europe. Life is about the ups and downs, the joys and challenges, the laughter and the tears. While our time in Lisbon was amazing, it wasn't without challenges. My husband's medical condition made it very difficult for him to constantly climb hills—hills that would present a great cardio workout for any healthy person. When climbing, I would walk behind him, hands on his lower back, providing a bit of a turbo-boost to help conquer the steep incline. The effort of walking on this hilly terrain, the initial challenge with medical equipment, the need to have natural light in our rather dark and chilly home—all added to the isolation that made our European transition longer and more difficult than expected.

Our angst quickly became evident during a Facetime with our son. His family had already arrived in Lagoa, Portugal both in preparation for our arrival in Albufeira (twenty-five minutes from their abode) and to begin their extended time living in the Algarve, escaping the cold, dark Finland winter. As parents, we feel the need to put on a brave face for our children, even our adult children, not wanting to burden them with our struggles. Much as I tried, the brave face was quickly replaced with tears as I shared how overwhelmed I felt, and the deep concern I had over dad's downturn in wellness. By the end of the call, we made the decision had been made to have our daughter-in-law and oldest grandsons make the drive from Lagoa to Lisbon a few days later, load up their truck with Rob's medical supplies, and pick up a rental car to drive the three-hour distance with them back to Lagoa. I felt like a burden had been lifted.

Four days later found us meeting Crystal, Matthew, and Samuel at the Oceanarium in Lisbon so they could follow us through the narrow, winding, hilly streets to where we were staying. They were a sight for sore eyes, as my parents would say. How good it was to see them! However, it wasn't until we all arrived back in Lagoa that the full joy of finally seeing our European kids after almost two years fully soaked in.

I digress… Navigating the narrow Lisbon streets was no easy task in a large SUV suitable for transporting our son, daughter-in-law, and their six children! Needless to say, I was in awe of Crystal's ability to navigate the route. Parking was, of course, another issue. On the narrow streets, there was not much room for a vehicle that large to pull over without blocking the road. Speed and care in packing the truck were of the essence. Without delay, the four of us got to work loading twenty-one boxes—twenty-five pounds per box—of dialysis solution into the vehicle, and within thirty minutes, they were on their way back to Lagoa, us following behind a short time later. Words could not express how grateful we were.

As a family, we have never been city dwellers. While we have enjoyed living in large cities like Vancouver and Edmonton, our small city of approximately 220 thousand people feels just about right for us. This became rather evident as we drove out of Lisbon, across the spectacular Vasco da Gama Bridge—the longest bridge in Europe, measuring seventeen kilometres. It felt like we were leaving the big city and heading to the country. We breathed a collective sigh of relief. Still, looking from the bridge over the Tagus River, seeing the many fishing boats awaiting high tide, witnessing Lisbon fade in the rear view, I experienced surprising and varied emotions. True, we were on to the next stage of our journey—which I knew we were excited for—and yet unexpected challenges had cut our time in Lisbon short. This added a touch of sadness to the varied emotions I was feeling; had we failed already? Had we given up too soon? I didn't think so. As a planner, I continue to learn that plans change—and not always at our choosing. Life happens, and at times, the adventure we call life presents us with the unexpected—and that unexpected can turn out to be even better than the original plan.

The drive to Lagoa was quite lovely. We were seeing the Portugal we could not experience flying into a city, exploring it, and getting on a plane to the next destination. We chose, unintentionally, to take the no-toll road from Lisbon, adding an extra forty-five minutes to the journey. But we didn't mind—it was beautiful to see the farmlands, the small towns and villages, and people going about their daily lives.

Having a GPS in the car was a blessing. But when your final destination doesn't have a specific street address, no amount of shouting or swearing (by me, not my hubby) at the GPS did anything to get us there. We arrived in the town of Lagoa without a problem, but our kids were living in the country outside the city. Fortunately, we had our EU phone set up for Portugal and were able to text our *SOS* to the family. Within minutes, a longitude and latitude location was sent for the general area, with assurance that our grandkids would be waiting to direct us to their long, hidden driveway.

If you are a fan of *The Sound of Music*, you'll recall the point where the children were all hanging off trees, anxiously awaiting the arrival of their father. We had our own *Sound of Music* experience. As we rounded the final corner before arriving at our destination, before us were four of our grandkids, standing on the wall, waving their arms to let us know we had arrived. I will never forget how my heart just about burst with joy at seeing them. It was one of the most beautiful sights my eyes have beheld.

Once up the driveway and parked, we were accosted with the biggest hugs imaginable from all six kids and their mom (our son had not yet arrived). It was happiness personified!

The week we spent with the family in Lagoa was simply amazing. I was finally able to dedicate some time and space to reading, thinking, and doing my research, while Rob lavished in precious time with the grandkids. Together, we were able to reconnect with our family in such a special way. As I think back on that week, my heart still sings with joy at the moments we shared. I am reminded of a breath-taking sunrise shared with Gracie, our second-oldest grandchild. She loved getting up early to watch the sun rise, so we chose a morning to make the ascent to the rooftop terrace and were rewarded with a kaleidoscope of colour never to be forgotten.

Most days, we would head to the beach, exploring the caves, climbing over rocks, and jumping the waves with all six grandkids. Listening to them chatter away, sharing their many adventures, were times we treasured.

Crystal, our daughter-in-law, was always exploring the local area, looking for special places. One such discovery we shared was in Carvoeiro, a short seven-minute drive from their home. The walk took us along the most awe-inspiring cliffs overlooking the Atlantic, including a climb down to explore tunnels and cave lookouts. Amazing!

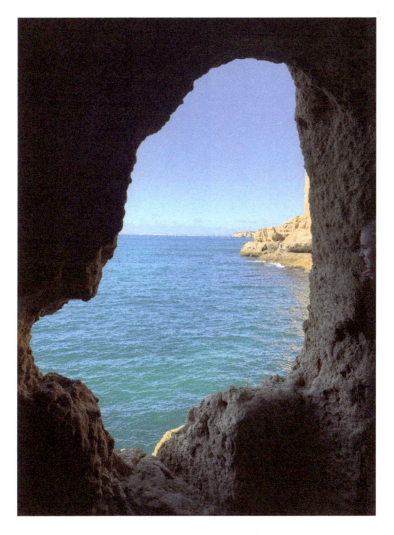

In the evenings, the living room fire would be lit to ward off the chill, and we would all sit around their big coffee table, enjoying a delicious supper prepared by Crystal or the kids. Papa would finish the day by reading a chapter from a favourite book, and eventually, everyone would mosey off to bed. Then, in the stillness, after all had gone to sleep, Rob and I would snuggle up on the big floor cushions in front of a roaring fire and reflect on our day or watch a favourite show on Netflix.

It was a week to remember.

CHAPTER 11

Leave home, leave the country, leave the familiar.
Only then can routine experience—buying bread, eating vegetables,
even saying hello—become new all over again.

—Anthony Doerr

We had left home exactly forty days before settling into Albufeira, Portugal. It felt like so much longer than that! It wasn't not a bad thing—just surprising.

After spending a great week with our family in Lagoa, we were ready to settle into our new apartment (I knew space was important to me, but I didn't quite realise *how much*). When we arrived, it was an overcast day. But when we walked into the third-floor apartment, we were immediately accosted by a spectacular view from the balcony. We could see the ocean! It had two bedrooms, a three-piece bathroom, a kitchen, an eating area, and a living area with two chairs, a couch, and a fireplace. Everything we needed. *And* the building had an elevator!

Our Albufeira abode offered a space where I could work from home. I could sit on the balcony and actually see the Atlantic, watching the sky take on beautiful hues as the sun rose and set, then cozy up at night in front of a real wood fire. This hadn't been the case in Lisbon—there, the need to go and do was strong, perhaps due in part to the lack of natural light (not even a window to look out!). Add to that the fact that we never conquered the chill that met us at the end of a glorious day exploring Old Town. I didn't feel inspired—or even welcome—in that apartment.

If you have ever moved to a new home, you may remember how the first few days you felt like a visitor, a guest. Not until you hung the pictures, put clothes in drawers and wardrobes, cooked a meal, made a pot of coffee, and really inhabited the house did it begin to feel like a home—a place that welcomed you when you walked in the door, kicked off your shoes, and put on your slippers. No matter how many meals, pots of coffee, or clothes unpacked, we never felt like more than guests in our Lisbon apartment. Contrast that to how we felt upon coming home to our Albufeira apartment: we felt settled, at home, and welcome.

For the next three months this *was* our home—close enough to the family for us to enjoy doing life with them, yet with our own space. We could do this!

While in Albufeira, there certainly were a few days where the reality of daily life was overwhelming, though. And I was sure more would come before our return to Canada. Just when I thought I'd come to terms with Rob's illness, a rogue wave of anguish would sneak up and slam me. Unfortunately, the way I dealt with such reality checks wasn't always positive or constructive. Perhaps this was the result of my being human. Or perhaps the outcome of my need to fix everything. I could not fix this.

Rob had been feeling unwell for the past few weeks (more so than his condition would normally dictate). Watching his decline created great angst for me (not to mention, for him as well!). After communications with his medical team in Canada, it was decided a video call was required. His nurse and dietitian came prepared for a conversation that was informed by a consultation with the nephrologist. Very quickly, the team observed that Rob was severely dehydrated, immediately prescribed an adjustment in his dialysis solution, and gently reprimanded for his low fluid intake. He was directed to go to a clinic in Albufeira, however, to see a doctor and have blood work done, just in case... (I hate 'just in case'!) He connected with an international clinic and saw a wonderful doctor who conducted a thorough examination. After several failed attempts to draw blood she made the decision that specialized laboratory technicians would be more successful at doing so.. Rob was directed to a lab where the doctor was sure they would have more success. We had no idea how challenging it was to take blood when a person was dehydrated! The wonderful nurses were just about in tears seeing the pain they were causing Rob. After twelve attempts, they finally had enough blood to run the labs. The results arrived later in the day, but it wasn't until the next morning that Rob had a conversation with the doctor. Spoiler alert... all was good, and the less desirable numbers would be addressed by the already-prescribed adjustments to his dialysis.

The point of this brief exposition is that as the days progressed until we were reassured that the symptoms were within the span of acceptability, my anxiety played out in irritability. Words from the song by the Mills Brothers came to mind: "You always hurt the one you love, the one you shouldn't hurt at all."

The day of the tests was also the first day of torrential rain in Albufeira—a much-needed rain. But the gloom didn't help my state of mind. The next morning, I knew I had to get outside, to the ocean—which I did. As I soaked in the freshness after the storm, delighted in the mist over the water, listened to the crash of waves and the screech of seagulls, and took in the mindboggling beauty of the place, the angst began to lift—just as the mist began to dissipate.

Loneliness and home sickness had been knocking on the door of my heart during such times. Being far away from our daughter, son-in-law, and granddaughter in Canada was hard, and we missed our friends terribly...virtual contact was just not the same as being physically present with those we love.

Trusting we were over the biggest hurdles of the trip, we happily adjusted to life in the Algarve. We enjoyed a simple routine. Mornings were spent mostly working on my research, afternoons on exploring, and then back to the research in the late afternoon and early evening, when I returned... mostly reading. In the evenings, we would light a fire and watch Netflix or just chill with a book. It was a pretty simple life.

One of the reasons we had chosen to spend time in Albufeira was to be by the ocean, and I thoroughly enjoyed it. We spent a great deal of time walking on the beach... it was massive! It truly was a place of healing—a place where emotions brimmed to the surface with such force, they couldn't be ignored. Being at the ocean has always brought me a sense of peace. However, the emotion revealed on one particular day was wrought with anything but peace, rather a release of pent-up anxiety that was stopping me from finally accepting that life as we knew it was no more. We had to find a new 'us', re-commit to creating new memories. It was so challenging!

We were not in Europe for a vacation—I was there to work. I was being paid to do this research. One of the downsides to my strong work ethic was a feeling of obligation to produce results, to justify the investment the college was making in me. A need to be doing. This drive was preventing me from learning, from slowing down enough to focus on the plan I had laid out... a plan that called for time to reflect.

Once we had settled in Albufeira, I finally revisited my learning itinerary, refocused, and got past the guilt of not always *doing* something research- or work-related. I was then able to slow down and enjoy time. It was good to review the transcripts from all my interviews and think about what I had heard. I also did more reading, intentionally taking time to ponder what authors were saying. I was finally physically slowing down. I remember feeling my head also slowing down and being able to process what I was learning. Rather than having focus, my headspace had felt more like driving on the 401 in Toronto, Canada (the busiest highway in the world). Before this slowing down, I would read material and have no idea what I read five minutes previous… *crazy*.

Finding a regular café to work from had not yet happened, in either Lisbon or Albufeira. To be fair, I am rather picky about what I look for in a location from which to work. My criteria: good coffee (important when you only drink decaf!), a strong Internet connection, and an atmosphere where you feel welcome to spend a couple hours working. If the space is not visually stimulating, I need a view. I also like when others are enjoying the café. There's something comforting about the buzz of conversation among those wrapped up in a shared experience.

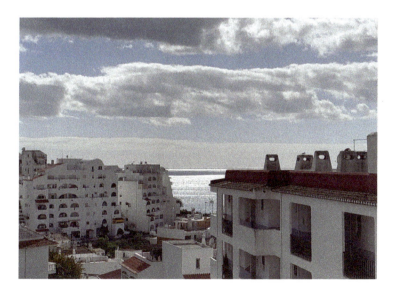

The view from our balcony in Albufeira

However, sitting out on the balcony of our home was great, so for work that called for the Internet, I stuck to home. For reading books, I made my way to the beach, where I could read, then think, then read. The other aspect I kept overlooking was the actual experience of travelling and working. All we were experiencing—good and bad, challenging and rewarding, funny and sad, lonely and comforting—was part of the learning journey. Working remote, whether full or part time, inevitably integrates life with work, and it's not always the fairy tale life many paint it to be. Rather, it takes discipline, self-management, self-leadership, an ability to adapt, and a huge dose of curiosity.

CHAPTER 12

It's not what's under the Christmas tree that matters, it's who's around it.
—Charles M. Schulz

On the first of December, 2021, the Christmas music was streaming on my computer. That's the way we've always done it. December first marks our son's birthday and the official start of the Christmas season. Some traditions travel with you no matter where you are. But travel also presents the opportunity to adopt new traditions. I was curious to see which ones we would take home with us to Canada at the end of our sojourns.

I don't love snow, but there is something about Christmas that brings with it a heart- warming, fairy tale image of tobogganing down hills, gently falling snowflakes, chestnuts roasting on an open fire, Jack Frost nipping at your nose… OK, let's not get carried away. I lived in Ireland until I was twelve… not much snow or tobogganing happening there. But Canada was home, now—and such an idyllic Christmas season is always a real possibility.

Over the years, the Christmas season has become increasingly commercialised, but my stomach still flutters when I think of the magic and meaning behind it. Once December arrives, our home is filled with Christmas music—both current songs and age-old carols. I love thinking of what gifts would be most meaningful for those special people in my life. I love the lights and the joy decorations bring to young and old alike. I love the time spent with family and friends—and the mouth-watering Christmas baking they do (I'm not much of a baker). My favourite has always been chocolate fudge shortbread, a treat my mum used to make that has now become our daughter's specialty.

Christmas 2021 was different… very different. My dad passed away in 2021. (Remember one of my what-ifs was my dad passing away while we were gone? As it turned out, he passed away in July—and I was blessed to be by his side as he slipped away.) COVID very much dictated what holiday traditions could be enjoyed—and which ones were quickly becoming memories from Christmases past. We were not in Canada, nor were we able to be with dear friends. And we deeply missed our daughter and her family.

However, the sweet memories of Christmases past were ever present in our hearts and minds. This year was a time to make new memories.

I remember one of my first beach walks in Albufeira. That was a true novelty for me—no need for winter jackets, gloves, toques, or boots. No snow. Most days, the sun shone, but even on cloudy or rainy days, the weather was very mild.

Rather than the crunching of glistening snow, my feet sank into the soft sand as I revelled in the majesty of the glistening Atlantic Ocean, while the sun sparkled on the white caps. Watching the mist clear after a storm was truly a sight to behold.

But the pièce de résistance was that we got to spend Christmas with our son, daughter-in-law, and six grandkids. What a treat! The times we have been blessed to share Christmas since their move to Europe are also embedded in our bank of never-to-be-forgotten moments. Over the previous years, we had spent two special Christmases with them—one in Ireland and one in France. Now, we got to add Portugal to the list. Papa and Gramma were truly blessed to share their home over this wonderful holiday time.

The excitement grew as the days approached. The thoughtful planning of how we would spend our time: the games we'd play, movies we would watch, and, last but not least, what yummy food we would prepare and enjoy. To top it off, Gramma would be joining in their Christmas Day tradition of jumping into whatever body of water they happened to be living on. So glad they were spending those few months in Portugal, away from the frigid Baltic Sea by their home in Finland!

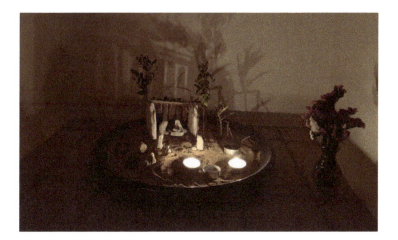

Christmas was wonderful. Our six grandkids (now aged nine through eighteen) lovingly created decorations—the quality of which equalled anything in a Christmas magazine—and displayed them with pride. On Christmas Eve, the children put on their traditional Christmas play… *oh my*! Our grandparent hearts just about exploded with joy, pride, and amazement at their dedication and creativity in re-enacting the story of

Christmas in song and spoken word. One grandson even saved some of his dad's beard shavings (Nathan has quite the Viking beard) and pasted them on his face to be more "authentic" in his depiction of a shepherd. We were doubled over in laughter when he turned to face the audience to reveal his transformation.

Our Christmas Day dip was indeed refreshing. The water wasn't cold, nor was the air, adding to the experience. I was, however, taken by surprise by the strength of the waves and the undertow. My assumption that all the hill-walking and stair-climbing of Lisbon and Albufeira would rebuild my strength after knee replacement was mistaken. How wonderful to be able to grab the hand of my grandson as I struggled to gain my balance and unstick my feet from the sinking sand as the tide fought against itself.

Crystal home schools the kids, and they blow me away with how much they know about… well… everything! I think it's fair to say travel is an education in itself, but combining that with intentional learning about the history and geography of where you are living, and it's unequalled. What could be better than learning about the history of Rome while camping just outside the great city, or studying design while living in the Netherlands, or learning about ocean tides while living by vast bodies of water in Ireland, Portugal, or Spain?

It is fascinating being in a culture so different from your own for such a significant and tradition-filled season of the year. Significant, from my perspective. I expected a similar celebratory atmosphere in Portugal as we had in Canada. Or that I had as a child in Ireland. I expected decorations that celebrated both the sacred and secular expressions of the season in homes and shared spaces. There were some, but they were minimal at best. But it felt like one could easily miss the fact that it was Christmas.

In the centre of Old Town, there were a few booths selling mulled wine and other Portuguese treats, though, and there was even a large tent set up with an ice-skating rink. Live Christmas music was performed on some evenings, with a small number of people partaking in the offerings. From an outsiders' perspective, it didn't feel like a community coming together to celebrate. I would like to have known and experienced whatever it was this culture held as significant and precious during that Christmas season.

It was raining on the evening before Christmas Eve. Where else would an Irish-born woman go on such a rainy day but the pub? The Guinness and warm Irish whisky were a true tonic for the deep cold that came with the rain and incredibly high humidity we experienced during those days. The owner had planned to celebrate with patrons throughout the season, until the announcement of new restrictions to curtail the spread of the new COVID variant. The plug had been pulled, so to speak, on their ability to facilitate festivities.

How realistic were my expectations? Was what I was observing normal for the area, or had people already dialled back their celebrations in response to the pandemic? Questions I never really got answers to. However, no matter what the world around us was doing, our Christmas was everything I hoped it would be.

CHAPTER 13

*You are never too old to set another goal
or to dream a new dream.*

—C. S. Lewis

It was Sunday evening, church services were done, and the sitting room was all set up ready for company. Mum had been preparing for our visitors over the past couple of days, and the spread she presented was nothing short of cookbook-front-cover-ready. The sandwiches were trimmed and cut into triangles, the scones were the perfect three-bite size, ready to be lathered with Devonshire cream and homemade strawberry jam. Mince tarts, chocolate fudge shortbread, plain shortbread, and Victoria sponge cake were all part of the fare, served on a triple-layer cake plate. Now, with the fireplace blazing, the room provided a warm and welcoming atmosphere for some good Irish craic with friends.

If you think Mum put on this spread for a special occasion, you'd be greatly mistaken; this was an entertaining norm for a family in Northern Ireland, right up to when we immigrated to Canada in 1970. People would feel free to drop in anytime, knowing the kettle was boiled, ready to "wet the tea" and let it "draw" for the appropriate amount of time. And the pantry always had a tea treat at the ready for those who dropped in.

This was our habit each Sunday evening. We enjoyed similar times at my grandparents' home in Annalong, too. I have fond memories of sitting around the fire, listening to my Granda recite stories and poems from years gone by in his gentle Irish brogue while Granny cooked up her delicious tomato soup in the tiniest kitchen possible (I've no idea how they raised six boys in that tiny home!).

When our family immigrated to Canada, we expected those cultural habits to continue for us. Dad and Mum expected neighbours to drop by anytime for a visit, and they expected Sunday evenings after church to be times of getting together with new friends. Sure, my parents still invited people over, and guests were delighted by the table spread before them (with a greatly reduced salary, the fare was simpler, but every bit as delicious), but such visits only happened when intentionally planned for. No one dropped by for a cup of tea. Mum waited, but no knocks ever sounded on the front door. It didn't take long before her confidence started to crack. Did people not like her? Was she an inadequate hostess? Would she ever have close friends again? It was a devastating turn of events for her, an accomplished homemaker who freely expressed her love and appreciation for others through hospitality.

Culture was not a topic of conversation back then. People were people. We didn't encounter folks from other countries on our small island (the cultural landscape of Ireland has certainly changed over the years... a lovely thing to see). In our new home, we knew things were different, but had no words to describe it—only expressions of sadness, hurt, and longing for what had been.

Eventually, after suffering a heart attack, my dad met an Irish doctor, who opened our eyes to the 'Canadian way'. Doctor Mark quickly became a family friend and provided our first lessons in Canadian culture. Who would have thought it would be considered an imposition to drop in for a visit? We also learned that while our hot beverage of choice was tea, most Canadians enjoyed coffee, however, their intake was nowhere close to our daily consumption of tea. Our habit was to have tea first thing in the morning, mid-morning, before going to the market, when we came home from the market, with lunch, in the afternoon, at dinner, and, of course, at supper (the snack we had just before bed). Not until my then-boyfriend (now-husband) came into the family did we realise this was not the norm.

Culture is a beautiful thing, but some cultural practices or habits can be a barrier to fully enjoying the many wonders of life. Let me share an example. As a young woman, I suffered from constant headaches. I saw one specialist after another, and none of their brilliant minds could figure out the problem. Until one. This doctor was an eye, ear, nose and throat specialist. But most significant was his heritage: he was British. In our first consultation, he inquired about my tea-drinking habits. When I recounted a normal day, we added up how many cups of tea I was consuming… more than ten cups a day, well beyond the recommended daily allowance of caffeine! His prescription was for me to stop drinking tea for a certain amount of time. I did and missed the tea desperately, but I did not miss the headaches that magically disappeared at the same time.

Growing up, I had had no exposure to other cultures. Our family travels had mostly been to the South of Ireland, England, Scotland, Wales, and Canada. But there is a great difference between visiting a place and residing in one. Merriam-Webster offers this as a definition of the verb *to reside*: "to be present as an element or quality." I certainly hoped being in a place for four months—as we were in Portugal, then Spain—would afford us true cultural insight.

We were not disappointed. Sitting at a cafe, on the beach, sipping some delicious Portuguese wine, my husband and I had a great discussion about the cultural differences we were observing between Portugal and Canada. We laughed. The very fact we had been sitting, sipping, for over two hours, with no one hovering, wondering when we would leave—no server coming to offer the *conta* or asking if we wanted anything else—was a stark contrast to what we would have experienced at home. In fact, I had recently booked a table for dinner at a Kelowna restaurant and received immediate notice it was ours for two hours maximum!

Portuguese people know how to relax and truly enjoy the moment. No one is in a hurry (even if you really had to leave a restaurant for an appointment!). We simply learned to ask for the bill quite a while before we needed to leave. It truly was a joy to have had such a minimal schedule, so that waiting to pay was not often an issue.

There were a few other differences we took note of. In North America, we take pride in providing clear directions and expectations—at times, to the point of over-explaining. However, we found that folks in Portugal offered broader explanations with limited detail, expecting you to fill in the gaps. On our first day in Albufeira, we asked for directions to a *pastelaria* (a pastry shop). We were told by our accommodation host that one was just up the hill and around the corner. Easy, right? Not so. Walking was complicated enough, but the directions failed to mention the number of one-way streets we'd encounter endeavouring to drive there. From my readings, I learned this communication difference was referred to as the difference between "high-context" and "low-context" cultures. A high-context culture, like that of Portugal, expects one to fill in the gaps and read between the lines, and a low-context culture, such as North America's, calls for everything to be stated—no room for ambiguity.

Another interesting observation related to when places were open or closed. Because of the time of year in Albufeira, many places were simply closed until the arrival of tourists sometime around the end of February. *When* in February? Well, that was rather vague. Many places were already closed when we arrived in November, with either no signage indicating when they would re-open, or a sign simply stating that they were closed for the holidays. Some opened for two weeks around Christmas, then closed again at the end of the first week of January, when they were once more *closed for the holidays*. Apparently, holidays could be four months, two weeks, or even five days a week.

One place we kept trying to go for Sunday pot roast turned out to be quite a challenge. The first time we went, most menu items were not available due to restrictions that required them to limit patrons for a number of days before Christmas until after the New Year. The second time we went, arriving for dinner at four-thirty, we were told they only served food until four. No problem, we would come back next Sunday for their special pot roast, or roast chicken dinner, served from noon to four. The day came, and my husband was pumped! He was salivating over the prospect of Yorkshire puddings. We arrived, sat down, and were quickly told the cook had decided to take the week off, so they weren't serving food that week. *Really*?! At this point, it became laughable. Even the British proprietor had been influenced by the Portuguese culture they had been part of for so many years. Seeing our disappointment and what-can-you-do laugh, they assured us that next Sunday, pot roast would be served up, guaranteed. The following Sunday, we were there at three for the much-anticipated roast meal, snatching the last table available.

The meal came, and it was rather delicious and very generous. But I felt cheated. Not because of the quality of food—or the generous quantity of it —but because I was in Portugal, eating a traditional English Sunday lunch, drinking Guinness, surrounded by British people. I missed hearing a cacophony of conversation in multiple languages, eating food whose ingredients I couldn't quite guess. Even trying to guess what was in the food brought back a lovely memory of my Granda famously asking my Granny 'What's in tilt, Daisy?' when enjoying one of her delicious homemade Irish meals. After this British Pub lunch, we decided to frequent restaurants featuring local cuisine, offering a more culturally relevant experience.

We quickly learned that buying food for a week, as we were accustomed to at home in Canada, didn't work in Portugal. When you buy fresh without preservatives, the produce simply doesn't last as long (but was it ever tasty!). Going to the market became a regular activity. I'm not a shy person, but it was a challenge to be aggressive enough to have the produce guy notice me—apparently, it wasn't impolite to elbow yourself in to get what you were looking for. I just had to learn the system, and all was good. And while going to the butcher three times a week with my Mum in Ireland had been easy, trying to figure out how to ask for lamb to be cut up for stew, or meat to be ground for chilli posed quite a challenge when I couldn't speak Portuguese, and the butcher couldn't speak or understand a word or English. At first it was very frustrating, but then, quite fun! I learned the Portuguese words for what I wanted and would be thrilled when they indicated they would cut it the way I asked.

We also learned that private conversations were public conversations. While sitting on our balcony, we would hear folks in the parking lot shouting up to their buddies… no matter the time of day (or night!) or the topic at hand. It was fun once we got accustomed to it.

And did you know that sidewalks aren't just for people? No—they are also for cars if they can't find anywhere else to park. And wine or beer is a great idea for a morning coffee break—or even for breakfast! It's true. It was amusing to see a couple of older *avós* (grandmas) each enjoying a refreshing beer with their breakfast at 9 a.m.

At the start of our preparations for travel, I had been frustrated dealing with the Portuguese consulate. Seven months later, I gained a greater understanding of the culture. I would have been well advised to take time to learn more about it before embarking on our journey. As part of my research, I read Erin Meyer's *The Culture Map*.[3] I devoured it! Its insights not only helped me grasp differences from culture to culture but also greatly increased my appreciation for them. To say my curiosity was sharpened would be an understatement.

One of the beauties of Europe is that just about everywhere you go, you will encounter folks from many cultures. Just be quiet and listen to the languages being spoken. For us, it was intimidating and exciting at once. There was such a beauty to it. Fortunately, the majority of people in Portugal spoke some degree of English (how I wish I had learned a second language!). One day, we were enjoying breakfast at a cafe by Oura Beach in Albufeira. Over the course of our meal, we visited with other customers, some short-term visitors, others more long-term hailing from Ireland, England, Wales, Germany, India, and of course, Portugal. It was so much fun. The common thread, of course, was travel—and a love for learning about others' experiences.

Later that week, my husband and I drove to the end of the world, Sagres. At least, that's what Europeans considered it until the fifteenth century. Sagres is a small village of two thousand people, located on the very southwestern tip of Portugal, and is a place like no other we have experienced. A small town, its beauty is truly beyond words, from the landscape to the hundred-plus species of flora, to the cliffside paths overlooking the unending ocean, to the twenty-five isolated beaches full of avid surfers. And of course, we can't forget the fearless line-fishing

---

3   Erin Meyer, *The Culture Map: Breaking Through the Invisible Boundaries of Global Business* (PublicAffairs, 2014).

happening on the precipice of 200-foot-high cliffs! It truly blew my mind. Did these people not know the certain death they were inches away from? Well, apparently, they did. But it hadn't curtailed those brave souls from fishing there for many years. Those were some of the sights that reminded me I was from Canada... our authorities would have shut such activity down because of potential danger. I lost count of how many times throughout our travels we commented on how restrictive North America is when it comes to potential personal harm.... apparently, we North Americans need someone else to let us know what is dangerous, and set up rules to save us from ourselves.

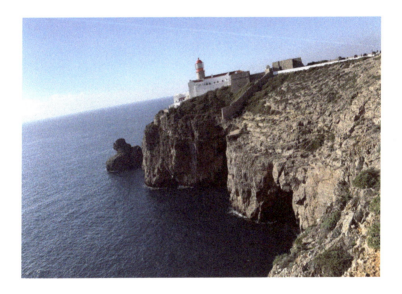

Sagres, the end of the world

I digress.... While walking around the peaceful Fortaleza de Sagres, we passed a lovely elderly couple who were clearly enjoying their time exploring the area together. By the third time our paths crossed, it seemed right we should have some kind of interaction. We exchanged greetings, though neither of them spoke English.

We learned they were from France. When we said we were from Canada, they immediately assumed we also spoke French. They excitedly named some of the places they had visited: Montreal, Quebec City, Montcalm, and Gatineau, to name a few—places I had also visited. However, when we somehow communicated that we were from the West Coast of Canada and couldn't speak a word of French, they offered a rather sympathetic "Vous ne parlez pas français aussi?" (You do not speak French either?). Still, using body language and simple words, we were able to share a moment together celebrating the awesomeness of the surrounding creation that had enraptured us. We said *au revoir*, they said goodbye, and we parted ways. But that short encounter brought certain joy— these fellow travellers had a deep appreciation not only for our similarities, but also our differences.

Taking a moment here to reflect on my research, the idea of *culture being habit* shifted my mindset over the course of my learning. "Organisation culture" or "team culture" is a topic of great interest in these changing times. We read articles and books about adapting to culture, learning a culture, creating a culture, or embracing a culture, among other topics, but the challenge seems to be most apparent when we start looking at *changing* culture. After reading this quote by Jutta Eckstein and John Buck I was challenged to look at culture through a different lens:

> "Culture will not change by propagating different values. Culture can only change by changing habits and behaviours. These, in turn, will change values, plans, procedures, and norms, and finally, the 'stories we tell ourselves about ourselves' regarding our bottom-line assumptions and beliefs."[4]

---

4 "Changing the culture by changing habits." Agile Today, accessed April 10, 2023, https://www.agileaus.com.au/changing-the-culture-by-changing-habits/

While changing my behaviour around drinking copious amounts of tea may not revolutionise an organisation, it was a change in my habits—my culture—that certainly brought healing and relief from crippling headaches. It freed me to more fully enjoy life (and opened up the whole new world of coffee—decaf, of course!).

As February dawned on us, we were reminded that our time in Albufeira was quickly coming to an end. What did we still want to do? What places did we want to revisit? What had we learned? Our one disappointment with Albufeira had been that it had been lacking in life while we were there. Many stores, restaurants, and businesses were closed—some due to the season, but others due to COVID. This made it quieter than we had expected, and at times, certain areas seemed deserted. We certainly couldn't complain about having the beaches to ourselves, though. That doesn't happen often, and we truly treated it like our own backyard. Nothing could take away from the beauty we had all around us, and the great workout we got from simply walking around the area of the Old Town.

CHAPTER 14

The cure for anything is salt water: sweat, tears or the sea.
—Karen Blixen

I love the sea—just ask my family and friends. Not simply enjoying a seaside vacation, playing in the sand, or jumping waves. My love for the sea is so deeply rooted in my psyche, it's hard to put into words. I love the smells, sounds, sights, and the feeling of sea salt on my lips and skin. Every chance I can, I head to the ocean. It's my happy place—my go-to when life gets overwhelming or doesn't make sense. Being by or on the sea brings forth certain emotions—a visceral reaction every time I get to be in its presence—an inner peace, an awesome appreciation. It's why I choose to spend eight months in Portugal and Spain—by the ocean.

I grew up by the sea in a beautiful town called Bangor in Northern Ireland and loved to visit our grandparents an hour down the coast in Annalong, a small fishing village. What I loved about both places was the location… right on the Irish Sea. My Uncle Artie was a fisherman. His "office" was a fishing vessel on the wild Irish Sea, an area notorious for having some of the roughest seas around Britain. Our family vacations, whether in the South of Ireland, England, Scotland, or Ibiza, were always by the sea.

One day while in Albufeira, we had an amazing experience that added to my rich bank of memories of adventure on the sea. The adventure was all about sailing on the Atlantic, looking at the shores and mighty cliffs of the Algarve. To celebrate our fourth grandchild's thirteenth birthday, the ten of us joined with eight other travellers for a three-hour expedition in search of dolphins (which, to our delight, we found!), then to cruise the coastline to marvel at the caves and spectacular beaches, many of which are only accessible by water. Though it was a rather cool, damp day (very Irish), the experience was magnificent and exhilarating. I felt a feeling of wonder and insignificance in the vast body of water, and deep peace and contentment. It was one of those transcendent moments.

Perhaps because I grew up by the sea, I have a healthy respect for the power it holds and the need for warning signs to guide ships and small vessels to safety. Warnings that can be relied on, warnings that are constant. Warning signs that, if ignored, can end in catastrophe.

My uncle knew what to look when avoiding danger on those days when the swell of the water threatened to swallow the vessel. Before the GPS was created in the late 1970s, fishermen like my uncle depended on the beacon of a lighthouse to guide them to shore, keeping them from being dashed on treacherous coastlines. They knew they could trust the lighthouse—that it was reliable, constant, a lifeline to guide them into the safety of the harbour.

As my research continued to focus on leading in uncharted waters, I wondered what warning signs might be ignored by men and women who care deeply about those they lead. I wondered if perhaps, in their desire to feed and nurture others, they become too busy to notice their own needs, only to find themselves dangerously close to the rocky shoreline, having ignored their own warning signs.

Two more weeks in Albufeira before we headed to Valencia, Spain. We were thoroughly enjoying the balmy weather, the azure skies, sometimes dotted with fluffy clouds and the occasional refreshing rain. Most days started with breakfast on the deck, where we could look out between buildings and clearly see the ocean spread out before us. The background sounds were made up of the squawks of seagulls, the sweet songs of various birds, people calling to each other on the street or from their balconies, and vehicles manoeuvring through steep, winding streets. The morning routine of hanging laundry out to dry and walking your garbage to the end of the street was embraced by all. Mail was delivered by a delivery person often driving a scooter, with parcels dropped off by the delivery van. Around ten each morning an elderly couple would walk down the hill for their morning coffee while locals gathered outside the cafe for a morning espresso and chat. All this from my office balcony perch on our fourth-floor apartment!

Some days, I headed to my favourite cafe, Roca Beach Bar, right on the beach. Yes, I had finally found an amazing place to work from. It took a couple of weeks, but what a treasure it was. Not only was the coffee good, but the *pastéis de nata* were amazing, served warm with cinnamon to sprinkle on top. I became a regular and received a warm greeting each time from the servers, and a genuine check-in to see how my work was going. They even designated a table as "mine"—one that welcomed me with an unobstructed view of the vast ocean just steps away. I loved watching people as they took their first walk along the beach. The awe and wonder on their faces was undeniable. I wanted to go to them and say, "Isn't this marvellous? Isn't it breathtaking?" But I didn't. With all the different languages we heard around us, chances were pretty strong that they wouldn't understand anything I said. Instead, we shared the unspoken nods, glances, and smiles that seemed to say everything.

Then, one day, the unexpected happened. Around five in the afternoon, the sun had lost its warmth and slowly slipped from view, eventually causing the air to drop to single-digit temperatures. I had no idea how cold it would be in the evenings in the south of Portugal. OK, not as cold as at home, but still cold. We learned the buildings were constructed to provide shade in the blistering summer heat, but were in no way equipped to warm their inhabitants during the winter. From the white concrete walls to beautifully tiled floors, construction intended to keep dwellers cool in the summer didn't feel so great when trying to warm oneself while huddled around a fireplace. Once you strayed more than a few feet from its blaze, the chill quickly wrapped itself around you.

Finding wood for a fire was easy in Albufeira; you simply added it to your grocery list and picked it up with your regular staples. *Oat milk, granola, eggs, fire starter, logs, firewood. Easy.* Except those nine-kilo-plus bundles were stacked in bins that require one to bend over, lift, twist, and drop into a shopping cart. I had been doing it successfully for two and a half months, until that day... the day the proverbial rubber band snapped. I have no idea what I did differently, except that my back decided enough was enough, and *snap*! Instant pain, instant "I can hardly move!," instant inconvenience. The shopping cart became my crutch until I reached the comfort of our car.

With the aid of a heating pad, topical cream, Tylenol, and rest, I got on my way to healing. The days following the snap certainly made getting comfortable a real challenge. Sitting for too long hurt, lying down made me ache, and my walking pace dropped a few gears, into slow motion. Though I knew the bricks in the footpaths had gaping cracks, the roads had many potholes, the stairs characteristically uneven, and the walk to the beach was a downhill trek (not to mention the uphill return climb), the pain that shot through my back with each crack, dip, and step drew attention to these irregular surface conditions. Nothing changed about the footpaths, roads, or hills, but my body had broken down, making it difficult for me to make do with the uneven terrain.

I obviously could not do anything to change the surface conditions in Albufeira, nor could I change the building construction; however, my rubber-band experience served as a reminder to pay attention to what I *could* change (like how I lifted things).

It got me thinking about life and work in general. When things are going well, when there are no new challenges to disrupt our flow, we don't pay much attention to minor inconveniences. Sure, they exist, but we work around them. We put up with them—until we can't. Why is it that an incident—be it catastrophic or minor—has to happen before we pay attention to those things we can change in order to make life better? Why do we settle for mediocrity when we could implement changes that could bring growth to our personal and professional lives?

Where is your happy place? Where do you go to hit pause, to recalibrate? Where do you go to get life back in perspective, to find balance, to get grounded when those rubber-band moments show up uninvited? To reflect? What refreshes and rejuvenates you so that you can continue to be the person those around you draw on for encouragement, support, and leadership? I'm more than happy to share my sea with you… .

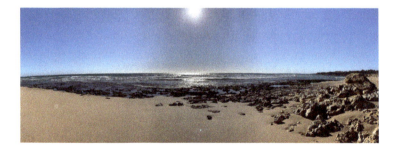

Praia da Oura Leste

CHAPTER 15

I have a theory about the human mind.
A brain is a lot like a computer.
It will only take so many facts,
and then it will go on overload and blow up.
—Erma Bombeck

I really love learning, but after a while, the research felt like a chore. I was mentally worn out. Growing up, if you were to ask my teachers or parents, they would not say a love of learning defined my school days—unless you were talking about anything to do with music. In high school, I had no problem getting to school by 7 a.m., three mornings a week, for choir and band practice, and I was thrilled to go to school on the days I had music classes in my timetable. But on the other days, I can't say I was a model student.

While I loved music classes at school, private piano lessons were a completely different thing. To be fair, my lesson followed my older, focused, and very musical brother. We both faithfully practised every day (thanks to Mum's perseverance), but somehow, Ian kept getting better; me, not so much. I still remember the horror of walking into a sterile, institutional building in Belfast to take a Royal Conservatory exam.

Then, the inevitable happened: our very stern piano teacher had a talk with my parents. It went something like this: "You are wasting your money having Roberta in piano lessons; she doesn't have a musical bone in her body." That was my last piano lesson. I was ecstatic! I now had an extra three hours every week to do what I loved—ride my bike, roller skate, and hang out with my friends. I wonder what Miss Thompson would say if she knew I went on to achieve first chair as a clarinettist in our high school orchestra and travel for two years in a prestigious singing group.

So, what made the difference in my musical education? I think two things were at play: a desire to learn about the subject matter and the learning environment. I really did *not* want to take piano lessons. I did, however, want to play the clarinet and sing. I love learning with others and have always loved creating music with others. And I never do well in a stick-and-carrot learning environment. It breaks my spirit and awakens my stubborn Irish ire.

Why was this concern over learning such a pervasive thought for me? What was irritating me? I had a desire to learn about the subject matter, and I was truly enjoying the experience of learning while in Europe. Still, if I loved learning so much, why was I feeling overwhelmed and fatigued? In one of my readings, I found this statement when reading a blog by Dean Yeong:

> "The abundance of information and the ease to access it quickly becomes a severe problem for people who are curious and want to learn almost anything. They're constantly consuming information to the point that they don't have the attention left to take action and to produce."

I wholly resonated with Yeong's sentiment. A fire hydrant of information was coming at me from every direction, too much for me to take in and learn from. This continues to be one of the disadvantages of ready access to the totality of human knowledge at our fingertips. This increased flow of information intake started during the previous two years. A total knee replacement quickly followed by COVID left me with more time to feast my curiosity. However, as with everything else in life, too much can lead to an overload. Add to that the emotional overload I was experiencing, and the makings of a perfect storm were present and accounted for.

As leaders, we are coached with such wisdom as Peter Drucker's belief that "learning is a lifelong process of keeping abreast of change. And the most pressing task is to teach people how to learn," or John F. Kennedy's opinion that "leadership and learning are indispensable to each other." Such appeals can unintentionally create added pressure, though. Don't get me wrong, I was committed to lifelong learning, I just needed to focus on what I could and should research in order to achieve my end goal—the purpose of the research.

I also realised my learning needed dialogue and debate with others who would challenge my thinking and shed light on the dark corners I was overlooking. I was missing that dialogue. The good news was I had amazing people in my life to call on: family, friends, and co-workers. But it was up to me to reach out to those I most respected and share what I was learning. It also was up to me to set up the necessary filters to prevent myself from drowning in an abundance of information and make time to consider what information was most valuable to what I truly cared about. But I also needed to give myself permission to hit pause, allowing the air to release from the overloaded balloon that was crushing my brain and emotions. I did. I put the books aside, shut off my computer, and rested my brain. Long walks with my husband, appreciating our surroundings, listening to music, and simply being, provided the pause I so desperately needed.

Once the pressure abated, I was ready to move on. When I read this quote by Peter Senge, it stirred my inner learner once again. This was why I was researching in the first place:

> *Real learning gets to the heart of what it means to be human. Through learning, we recreate ourselves. Through learning, we become able to do something we never were able to do. Through learning, we re-perceive the world and our relationship to it. Through learning, we extend our capacity to create, to be part of the generative process of life. There is within each of us a deep hunger for this type of learning.*

It was time to start writing about what I was learning, to get my thoughts onto paper and allow the process to help me sort through what was clear and what needed more clarity. If you had told me a few years previous that writing a paper would help my overloaded brain, I would have thought you rather daft. But that's exactly what happened.

With a renewed focus and commitment, the remainder of our time in Portugal was all about pulling together what I had learned, reflecting on what we had experienced, and preparing to move on to the second half of our time in Europe.

CHAPTER 16

*If you're brave enough to say goodbye,
life will reward you with a new hello.*

—Paulo Coelho

We first discovered Google Translate during our trip to Prague some years ago. It was amazing, and helped us out in so many ways, from reading menus to asking for directions. Our time in Portugal had also been aided by this helpful app. While most menus provided an English translation, we still had the need for language support in several other areas. Grocery shopping, for example, was an immediate area of challenge. The first day upon arrival in Lisbon, we needed to stock our little kitchen. No car? No problem. Grocery stores were within close walking distance from our Airbnb. For the most part, buying meat, cheese, fruits, and vegetables was easy (as long as one could identify what the fruit or veggie was). What wasn't so easy was knowing what kind of yogurt, oatmeal, milk, or even shampoo and conditioner was before us on the shelves. No problem, simply open Google Translate, use the camera feature, and we were good to go!

In one instance, while dining at a favourite Lisbon eatery, Basilio, there was a sign hanging on the basket of ginger on the counter by our table. The symbol was a dog sitting, with a line across the picture. We have similar types of signage in Canada to indicate such things as no smoking or no cell phones. You know the ones. Looking at the placement and location of the sign, we were certain the message was clear. My husband and I had a lengthy discussion about why ginger might be dangerous for dogs and why a restaurant would need to provide signage to that effect. Curious, and wanting to share this knowledge with family and friends, I took a picture. It wasn't until we returned to our apartment that I asked Google to translate the words accompanying the picture, "Nao sentar,"—"don't sit." Had we used Google in the restaurant, we would have learned this—but would have missed out on a very interesting conversation about the perils of ginger for our canine friends.

We had another incident where we wished Google Translate could have helped. In preparation for leaving Portugal for our new European location in Spain, we set out to return our small explore-the-Algarve vehicle in exchange for a larger one more conducive to the long drive from Albufeira to Valencia. We had originally planned to go vehicle-less while in Europe. While that is entirely possible in most places, we discovered travelling in the Algarve required one. There were so many places to visit and we did not want to miss out.

The new vehicle was to be picked up forty-five kilometres away, in Faro. After a rather frustrating experience with the car rental company, who had mistakenly reserved another small vehicle for us, we were upgraded to a Mercedes van—one they wanted to be returned to Spain after being dropped off by one-way travellers. It was big—larger than we needed or wanted. However, it provided comfort, and plenty of room for us, our luggage, and the medical supplies we were transporting.

My husband started the Mercedes and successfully drove out of the car lot, figured out where the gear changer was located, and headed back to Albufeira. Everything was good, until he touched a button or level, causing the car to get stuck in first gear. Finding a place to pull over, he pushed, tapped, and pulled on every available lever and button (of which there were many). We began to feel like our youngest granddaughter pushing buttons, pulling levers, and turning wheels to make things happen in her Fisher-Price car. The car was trying to tell us what to do by way of information showing up on the control panel. The trouble was, all instructions were in Spanish. Same with the car manual. There had been nothing in the basic Spanish lessons we had taken that had equipped us to get us out of this predicament, nor could our precious Google app get close to providing us with any kind of translation. Finally, after much random button- and lever-manoeuvring, the gear changer was released... though my husband had no idea which was had been the magic button.

Unsure of which road to take to get us home, rather than using my phone, I decided to use the GPS. I'm sure you can imagine what happened... everything was in Spanish. For my sanity's sake, I used my phone. Knowing we only spoke English, why no one at the rental place thought to introduce us to the machine we had just rented remains a mystery. But we stopped at one of their drop-off locations once we made it back to Albufeira, where a very kind service agent switched the system to English, linked my phone via Bluetooth, and introduced us to the various bells and whistles. We breathed a sigh of relief.

Both my husband and I are experienced drivers, having driven for more years than we would choose to mention. We have driven all kinds and sizes of cars, in various countries, but had never found ourselves in that kind of predicament. It's interesting how inadequate and foolish you can feel being confused and overwhelmed by something you have done for years. I have worked with leaders who felt like this. These folks had been leading teams successfully throughout their careers, but with the onslaught of a global pandemic, they had found themselves having to re-think and re-learn everything. They knew how to be effective, but what had once been familiar had changed. Learning how to lead and support their people in fast-changing contexts can be like operating a vehicle in an unfamiliar language, in an unfamiliar country.

Finally, our last day in Albufeira arrived—of course, it couldn't go by without one final walk along the incredible stretch of beach that had been our home for the past three months. There was not a breath of wind blowing, but the waves were still displaying their power for all to see. As I sat on the sand ridge created by the mighty ebb and flow of the water, I saw a big wave coming. I closed my eyes and listened… there was stillness, like the calm before a storm. Then came the crash of the wave, followed by the soaking I got as the ocean splashed over the sand ledge where I was perched. It drenched me and a couple sitting a few metres away. We looked at each other and laughed… what could you do? As the water receded, I heard the sound of shells rolling and soft, bubbling water as the next wave got ready to pound the beach. I could have listened for hours! The waterscape continued to change with every new wave. As we walked the beach on an almost-daily basis, we marvelled at how much it had changed—while still preserving its beauty.

Our time in Portugal had been fantastic. When I looked back at all I had accomplished over the previous months for research, I was amazed. At times, I had felt panicked, thinking I should be doing more, forgetting that sitting, thinking, and reflecting on what I had read or written was part of learning. But the four months we had spent in Portugal also provided us the opportunity to spend much quality time with our son, daughter-in-law, and grandkids. We dearly loved each of them and knew we would miss them terribly. In a way, though, it felt like we were venturing out on a new trip: new locations, language, surroundings, culture, living accommodation, food... new everything. We were excited.

As I sat soaked, in awe of such an amazing creation, my mind wandered. I used to think of the ocean, or sea, as being my happy place... I'm not sure that's still an accurate sentiment. Don't get me wrong: I will always love being by the water. But over those four months, it had become more than just my happy place. It had become a place where my thoughts found release, a place where I was forced to acknowledge that life can be shitty but *also* filled with joy. It's a place where I've been forced to come to terms with how I grew up viewing myself and where that negative thinking came from; where tough conversations had taken place, where words had been spoken from a place of hurt—words not totally seasoned with love and grace. It was also a place where long walks were enjoyed, hand in hand, with the person that I love more than life itself. It was a place where I paused to be vulnerable with myself and started learning to be brave enough to be vulnerable with others.

New memories had been created in Portugal that will stay with us forever: our Valentine's dinner watching the sunset over the Atlantic, lazy afternoons sipping wine and enjoying good conversation on the beach, mesmerised by the constant ebb and flow of the waves. The wonder at seeing how the beach and waterscape morphed over time, or watching an older gentleman make his frequent trips to the edge of the beach, stripping naked to thoroughly enjoy frolicking in the waves.

Before heading out on my final beach amble, I stopped at one of the cafés we had frequented to pick up a coffee and one last pastel de nata. You would think after four months of having them more often than I should, the novelty would have worn off... not so! Even now, as I dream of future trips to Portugal, I get excited about devouring those creamy custard delights.

At the time of our leaving, the area was starting to come alive again. When we had arrived a few months back, we had been told that late February to early March was when things started to fully open up—and they had been right. Two specific eateries we had been longing to visit finally opened; a café on a side street in Old Town and a lovely Italian restaurant whose menu had had us drooling. We treated ourselves two days in a row to their delicious offerings and were not disappointed. The café would have been a perfect place second place to work from… oh well, another time. I certainly can't complain about my café on the beach.

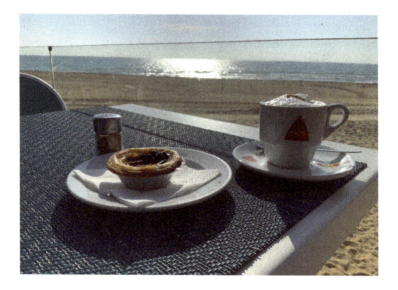

As I relished in my ruminating place, I noticed a deep sense of peace and contentment. I didn't want to leave. But I knew that without moving on, I would never experience the new, wonderful, and exciting adventures we had yet to encounter on our journey. *Spain, here we come!*

CHAPTER 17

It finally happened. I got the GPS lady so confused, she said, "In one-quarter mile, make a legal stop and ask directions."

—Robert Breault

Spain, here we are! From the peaceful, natural beauty of Portugal's Algarve to Spain's third-largest city, Valencia. What a change! The Algarve provided rest for my soul and a visual buffet for my senses, but Spain was different... so different. We had set out on this trip to experience new cultures, but never did I expect the culture shock that hit once we arrived in Spain. But I'm getting ahead of myself.

We left Albufeira at the end of February and drove to Seville, stayed for one night, drove to Torremolinos, stayed one night, and then drove to Valencia—all in a monster of a Mercedes van. Those of you living in North America may not get the magnitude of this task... let me paint a picture for you: two Canadians, used to driving a small SUV, driving a massive, seven-person van in the narrow, busy streets of Old Town Seville, depending on a GPS that kept getting them lost. It was not a task for the faint at heart. In fact, it was downright stressful. A fact to keep in mind: those narrow streets were one-way, so if you happened to miss the "obvious" turn Google was sure you needed to take, the recalculations took so much time that you would miss two or three more turns that would have taken you back to where you got lost in the first place.

Once we finally reached our destination, there was no place to park the van. But—thank goodness—we spotted a space that said something we decided to interpret as "only park here if you are checking into the Hotel Las Casas de la Juderia." We parked, and nonchalantly walked about fifty metres back to our hotel (our interpretation was pretty accurate!). After checking in, we took advantage of valet parking for an additional fee… money well spent. The wonderful valet whisked our car away and helped us with our mega-heavy luggage and medical supplies.

The hotel was amazing. The most unique one we have ever stayed in. Hotel Las Casas de la Juderia consisted of twenty-two restored eighteenth-century buildings, preserving its culture, furniture, and maze of hallways to navigate. It was located right in the middle of Barrio Santa Cruz. We only had a short time to spend in the amazing city, so we wanted to make the most of it.

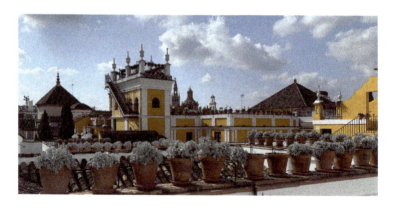

View from the roof of our hotel

After arriving mid-afternoon, we checked into our beautiful room (*that had a bathtub!*), unloaded our suitcases, set up medical equipment, and set out to explore. It was a warm, sunny day, and we welcomed being able to stretch our legs after a long drive. Our lunch had been consumed at a roadside restaurant, our first exposure to a dining establishment where no one spoke English and there was no English version of the menu. We were in Spain. This was clearly a new country—with a new language, new food, new culture. The server at our roadside stop was so gracious. Between pointing to others' meals, hand gestures, and of course, Google Translate, we ordered and enjoyed our meal, settled the bill, and paid more than we had for most of the meals we'd eaten in Portugal. Yes, we were now in Spain.

After wandering the quaint streets, browsing small stores, sampling the many sweets, liquors, wines, and sundry other things produced with Seville oranges, we were ready to sit and sip a glass of Spanish wine. Again, no English on the menu. However, we were able to discern the wine menu and ordered *dos copas de vino tinto*. Since we had already witnessed how displeased the server had been with a neighbouring table that only ordered drinks, we added an order of patatas bravas. This quickly became my favourite go-to for tapas. Refreshed and nourished, we were ready to see what was around the next corner.

While I'm a planner, I can be quite impulsive. When we rounded a corner in the Santa Cruz neighbourhood and saw a horse-drawn buggy for hire, I knew we needed to engage the driver. If you are short on time for exploring an area, I'd suggest this as a most delightful way to tour around, being regaled with stories about the history of the area by a buggy driver. We started at Real Alcázar de Sevilla and travelled through Maria Luisa Park, around the Plaza de Espana, past El Arenal, and everything in between. What a beautiful area, viewed in such a fun way!

The patisseries in Seville—and all through Spain—are a temptation that even the most disciplined among us would have a hard time resisting. I am disciplined, but not *that* much! Still not hungry after our wine and tapas, we decided to get a takeaway treat from a patisserie by our hotel in the San Bartolome area. I'm not sure what my husband ordered, but I do recall how they used such care in wrapping my decadent chocolate dessert in wax paper, tied with baker's string. I carried it back to our room with tender care—I didn't dare drop it.

Earlier, we had been fortunate enough to secure tickets to a flamenco show that night. I love Flamenco and was excited to take in a show in Seville! According to one travel site,[5] "Flamenco is surely the purest expression of Andalusian folklore. They say it began with the fifteenth-century arrival of the gipsies to the Cadiz countryside of Jerez and Seville. In the middle of the nineteenth century, it was popularised through the flamenco bars. The first of these flamenco bars opened in Seville around 1885."

If you have never experienced this spectacular dance, you must. The passion of the performers was something to behold—singers who put every part of their very being into the song, guitar players whose fingers moved so quickly and deftly one could easily be hypnotised, and the agility and power of the dancers...! Flamenco is one of those things you have to experience yourself. Words simply can't do it justice. At times, I had to remind myself to breathe—such was the connection between the performers and the audience.

After enjoying a much-needed sleep on an oh-so-wonderful mattress, our day began with a great buffet breakfast at the hotel.

---

5 "Getting to know the soul of a people," Seville City Office, accessed April 10,2023, https://www.visitasevilla.es/en/history/enjoy-flamenco-seville#:~:text=Flamenco%20is%20surely%20the%20purest%20expression%20of%20Andalusian,these%20flamenco%20bars%20opened%20in%20Seville%20around%201885.

All too soon, we were back in our giant vehicle, finding our way out of Barrio de Santa Cruz, through modern Seville, on to Torremolinos. The terrain was beautiful—so varied, with an abundance of olive groves that spread out as far as the eye could see. It was surreal when we saw the first direction sign for Africa as we approached Málaga. Africa will have to wait for another trip—another adventure.

We finally made it to our destination, where the GPS wrought havoc once more. When *the voice* said to turn right at the next turn, we figured it was safe to do so. Well, not when it was a dead-end street that ended in an underground parking lot with no way to turn around without heading into the bowels of the parkade! A one-floor basement parkade, with maybe fifteen parking spots fit for tiny cars and scooters. Again, my husband's driving skills were tested as I directed the inch-by-inch turn-around inside the parkade, back up the 12-percent-grade, spiralling road to the exit—which was also the entrance! Fortunately, no other vehicles decided to enter while we were trying to exit. Phew! Nerves shot, pulse racing, we made it.

Torremolinos is on the Mediterranean. I was so excited to be by the sea. Sadly, though, the weather was dull, overcast, and windy, so it did not show off its beauty. However, the next morning, it redeemed itself as the view from our hotel balcony provided a front-row seat to the sun coming up over the sea. *Lovely.*

After the most delectable breakfast I've ever devoured, champagne and all, we hopped in the van for the long drive to Valencia, where more challenges, adventures, and discoveries awaited us... along with culture shock.

CHAPTER 18

*A nation's culture resides in the hearts
and in the soul of its people.*

—Mahatma Gandhi

I hadn't been working on my memoir for a few weeks. Actually, not at all since arriving in Spain. I kept waiting for inspiration to write, like I kept waiting for the sun to shine. I have this thing about wanting to write about the good things—the amazing people and places we were discovering. The joys of travel and the new discoveries being made. But at that point in our journey, I was coming up blank. I think the first month in Spain will go down as the most challenging month of our entire time in Europe.

There were different things at play, including the heaviness of heart exacerbated by the poor weather and noise-disrupting sleep due to Fallas (a traditional celebration held annually in the city of Valencia in commemoration of Saint Joseph). However, the biggest issue was culture shock. I had heard about it, been aware of it, and downplayed it. But now, I was experiencing it. *Shock* is a great descriptor.

As noted earlier, when I was eleven my dad won an all-expense trip for the family to a location of his choosing for being the top salesperson in his company. My parents decided on Ibiza. It was truly amazing. The language was different and the food was unlike the meat, potato and vegetable meals we were accustomed to. I remember one dinner at the hotel in which we were staying. I can't recall what was on the menu, but whatever it was, our Irish tastebuds decided it called for ketchup. Admittedly, ketchup was like a side dish for us. Once the food was served, my brother naturally asked for ketchup. The look on the server's face removed any doubt that this was not customary for our chosen dish… or any dish served in the establishment. Still, he returned with the requested condiment—and the chef. They stood behind my brother and watched to see what he was going to do with the ketchup, then shook their heads and walked away. We thought this was funny, continued with our delicious meal, and decided that the Spanish people had strange ideas about food. We easily accepted it as being a cultural thing. No big deal. The language barrier, we overcame with non-verbal hand descriptions—aptly demonstrated by my dad—and learning very basic, important words and phrases: *baño, por favour, Cuánto cuesta este? Muchas gracias,* and, *Podemos tener más papel higiénico?* (can we have more toilet paper?). For two weeks, we were able to get by. We were also able to quickly adapt once realizing our mistake of remaining by the pool in the heat of the day. For two weeks we were able to get by.

A few decades later, I was once again in Spain. It wasn't so easy. We were not on vacation. It was not just about the sun or getting more toilet paper. We were not in the comfort of a resort. We were living in the old fisherman's quarter of El Barrio del Cabanyal. This area of Valencia was steeped in history. A walk around revealed glimpses of a turbulent past. It was a neighbourhood, not a tourist attraction. And English was not spoken by—well—*anyone*. For this, we were not prepared. It wasn't just the language. We felt like outsiders, like we didn't belong. We were not longed-for, welcome guests… we were trying to insert ourselves into someone else's home—and it was hard! Not only was the language different, the non-verbal actions were challenging to interpret. It was almost a feeling of indifference we were getting. Please don't misunderstand me—this was what *we* were seeing and feeling… it was not an exposé of the character or hospitality of the Spanish people. When we did find someone who could speak English, they were more than happy to help. The challenge was finding these people.

One experience that made our day took place at the market. We were stopping for lunch, and I wanted a croquette. The lady immediately started speaking Spanish at lightning speed, but very quickly realised we didn't understand a word of what she was saying. So, out came her phone and I watched her text as quickly as she spoke. She then handed me her phone to read; she had typed out the many kinds of croquettes she made, put it through Google Translate, and waited for me to read and point to which one I wanted. I could have hugged her!

Another surprise was the constant setting off of fireworks. According to Mario, our amazing tour guide on a walk through Old Town, Spaniards love fireworks—the noise, the smoke, the smell of gunpowder, everything. Now, I love a good fireworks display; growing up in Ireland, we celebrated Guy Fawkes Day with fireworks and huge bonfires. This wasn't that. It was early March when we arrived in Valencia… time for Las Fallas. Officially, the festival runs from the fifteenth of March through the nineteenth, with Noche de la Cremà, the evening when the Fallas are burned, finishing the celebration off. However, the locals start celebrating March first, with firecrackers going off every few seconds. I immediately had flashbacks to Northern Ireland, coming home from a holiday. As we left the airport and drove down a hill into Belfast, we saw several cars stopped, with drivers and passengers out of their cars, overlooking the city. We joined them. The noise of bomb blasts and flashes of lights from the explosions made such an impression on my young mind. The constant firecrackers in Valencia brought back the memory—and panic—as though it was yesterday. It certainly caught me off guard.

For those who enjoy an elevated *BOOM*, though, a thunderous firecracker show called la mascletà was held every afternoon at two in Plaza del Ayuntamiento. My husband attended, while I remained as far away as possible, by the Central Market. It was unbelievable. The ground literally shook under my feet!

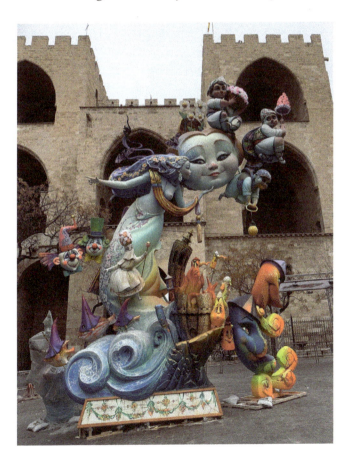

Torres de Serranos provided the background to one of the hundreds of Fallas

As we walked around our neighbourhood, we saw large groups of people celebrating together. It was like multiple block parties, with paella being cooked on open fires in the middle of the road, lots of laughter and drinking. We walked by, observing but not joining. We were outsiders, not part of their history, present, or future. It really was lovely to see the community created by these folks. It made me miss home.

One of my projects while on leave was to study for and write the exam for my GPHR (Global Professional in Human Resources) designation. The module I was studying at the time focused on culture—in particular, culture shock. The context related to organisations supporting expatriates going on assignment to other countries. As I read through the general symptoms, I was amazed at how many I was experiencing. The list included: irritation, homesickness, loneliness, nervousness, loss of appetite (not in my case), sleeplessness, feeling tired, extreme pride in one's home culture, hypersensitivity, and confusion. Pretty significant—and relevant. The good news was that, according to my study material, "culture shock is temporary, and everybody goes through it to some extent in the process of cultural adaptation."

Good to know. However, right then, the culture shock did not feel temporary. We were sojourners living in what seemed like a strange land. Every day things were fraught with difficulties—even finding a store within walking distance that would offer more than a basic convenience store did back home in Canada.

With so many people making the decision to work from anywhere, to mix work with travel, to relocate to a different country while working for someone in their home country, I am amazed by the lack of conversation about culture shock. When sending employees to work abroad, organisations need to take the responsibility of supporting and adequately preparing their people. But who prepares the individuals and families of those independent contractors and location-agnostic workers for such undertakings?

Let me strongly encourage those of you considering such a move to do your homework, take time to make informed decisions, learn the language, and make connections in your host country—and not underestimate the impact of culture shock.

When we eventually departed from Europe, we would have been there for seven months: Portugal for four and Spain for three. Our desire in Europe during this extended period was to experience and be part of the local culture. As we embarked on our journey, the plan had been to live in a local area—not tourist central. We wanted to learn what daily life was like, go grocery shopping, and cook most of our daily meals in our own kitchen. We wanted to learn which butcher was the best and which stand at the market had the freshest fruits and vegetables. We wanted to eat the local dishes and even learn to cook them. We wanted to wash our clothes in the small washing machines tucked under a shelf in the space-challenged kitchens, then hang them out to dry on clotheslines and balconies. We wanted to get a sense of the pace of life, and get to know which special occasions people in each location celebrated—and how they chose to celebrate. We wanted to take in the culture and arts scene and learn the history that brought each place to where they were now. All this we did—mission accomplished. But we also experienced an aspect of life we hadn't anticipated. We had felt it in Portugal, but it was even more evident in Spain.

The city of Valencia was home for a period of time, but we were not *at home*. We were neither tourists nor residents. We had friends come to visit… and leave. We stayed. We had a regular grocery store, doctor, medical lab, and transit pass (including Valenbisi, the city bike share), we paid electricity bills, had an EU phone number, knew the best local places to eat out, and even recognised regular local beach volleyball players. I had a membership at a local co-working space. We greeted many people but had no conversations (*no hablo Español*).

We didn't have friends or even acquaintances there. We were part of the city, but not part of the people. We contributed to the local economy but had no access to resident services (like a COVID booster). We couldn't access 1-800 numbers in Canada for things like travel insurance claims or queries about our TELUS phone bills. We observed the culture but were not part of it. I tried to search out expat communities and activities, with no success.

What were we? We felt somewhat displaced, like kids peeking through the hole in a fence to watch a party they weren't invited to. I shared these thoughts with some close friends back in Canada and felt my heart warmed by their encouraging words:

> You are a Canadian temporarily removed from those who miss you terribly and want you back where we can have face-to-face conversations. And drink wine. And taste some of the delicious foods that you want to make for us as we listen to your stories and share in the complex evolution of growth and perspectives.

It was an interesting state in which to find oneself. Please don't misunderstand—we were learning and experiencing so much. Our lives will be forever marked by that time abroad. But it was different than we had expected. Different than we had been prepared for. Our perspectives, opinions, and assumptions were challenged.

While we were both living the same experience, my husband's reaction was somewhat different than mine. He was content to be an observer—to watch, listen, and just be in the moment, taking in the sights and sounds. For me, I like to start by observing, but once I have a lay of the land, I want to jump in, be part of, and belong. But as an introvert, I needed to be *invited in*.

So, how did we navigate through this state of being? We decided in the two and a half months until our return to Canada, we would continue using our online programs to learn Spanish, dig into understanding as much of the culture as possible, watch bonfires, admire *ninots* that circle the *remates* that make up the Fallas monuments,[6] find the best Paella Valencia around, learn to make it, spend as much time as possible at the sea, and observe, respect, and take in all the Spanish culture had to offer. We would be richer because of it.

Good news: we made an amazing discovery... a grocery store just a fifteen-minute walk, or five-minute bike ride away. And it had everything—with multiple choices! We felt like kids in a candy store. They even had chips to make nachos (one of my favourite comfort foods). This was even more special since our place in Valencia actually had an oven! Ah, the small pleasures.

---

6 "Everything You Need To Know About Las Fallas Festival In Valencia, Spain," Brogan Abroad, accessed April 10, 2023, https://broganabroad.com/fallas-festival-valencia-guide/

CHAPTER 19

*No distance of place or lapse of time
can lessen the friendship of those who are
thoroughly persuaded of each other's worth.*

—Robert Southey

They said that it hardly ever rains in Valencia. They said that being in Valencia for Fallas was a fantastic experience.... Our first three weeks in Valencia didn't quite line up with what *they* said. In fact, since our arrival on the first of March, we had experienced a meagre two days of sun. The rest had been overcast, rainy, accompanied by some mighty powerful winds. Each day I looked expectantly at the ten-day forecast, only to be disappointed at the repeated pattern of rain-wind-cloud for the foreseeable future. When friends asked what the weather was like in Valencia, I compared it to growing up in Ireland or being in Vancouver in the fall. We never expected Spain to be this bone-chilling, windy, or grey. But eventually, there would be a light at the end of the tunnel, and it would look like a big, beautiful ball of fire in the sky... we hoped.

End of week four and yet another rainy day in Valencia. We had some lovely days the previous week and enjoyed them to the fullest. But the greatest reprieve came with the arrival of four of our good friends! Seeing them was like a breath of fresh air, like new life being breathed into us. How true are these words by Khalil Gibran?

In the sweetness of friendship, let there be laughter and sharing of pleasures. For in the dew of little things the heart finds its morning and is refreshed.

For a week, I closed my laptop, put aside my research and our efforts to be locals, and fully embraced being tourists... and did we ever enjoy it. If you have never taken on the challenge of being a tourist in your own town, I highly encourage it. You see things through different eyes and experience things you take for granted. Though we were still temporary newbies in Valencia, it did feel like we were, in a way, welcoming friends to our place, our city. However, along with what had become familiar to us, like buses and trams, walks, and favourite eateries, we explored and discovered new areas of Valencia together.

The first meal when our friends arrived was at Boa Beach restaurant in Cabanyal, close to our flat and where our friends were staying. We celebrated being together again with laughter, great food, excellent wine and beer, and catching up on each other's lives. Boa Beach provided the perfect environment for our reunion.

Experiencing the gastronomy of a location is important... so much culture is reflected in the food. Paella, the rice dish originating in Valencia, was so delicious. The traditional paella is made with chicken and rabbit, while an authentic alternative features seafood. We discovered the best way to enjoy it was to take a paella cooking class (a no-brainer after the carbonara cooking class my hubby and I had taken a couple of weeks prior). Monday morning, we hopped on the bus to a not-yet-explored

Mercat de Russafa, where we met our paella chef and hostess. After shopping for ingredients at the market, we headed to our culinary classroom for an experience we would remember for many years to come.

First step… make sangria and enjoy chef-prepared tapas. We were off to an amazing start. The chefs then took us step by step through the preparation process, explaining the history of paella, along with the essentials that go into creating an authentic one. The best part came when we all relished the fruits of our labour. This is a Valencia experience I highly recommend. A memorable aspect of the experience was meeting travellers from different parts of Europe—and even someone from Australia. The conversations were rich and energetic.

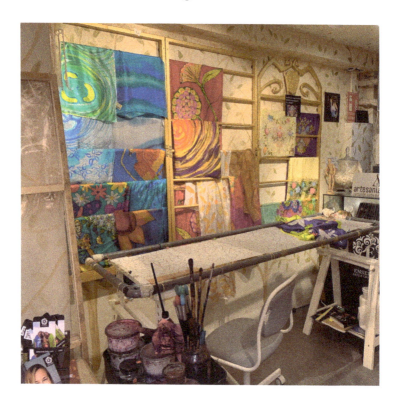

The next day, we found ourselves wandering Old Town, taking in the sights and sounds. We enjoyed lunch at a small tapas restaurant, prepared in a kitchen so small, no one could have imagined how delicious the food served from it could be. One of the treasures we found among the narrow streets of ornate, balcony-adorned buildings was a silk artisan. Her work was stunning—so much so, we just had to make some purchases. We were the first Canadian customers to purchase her work. What an honour for us to show off her work back home!

The remainder of the day allowed us to introduce our friends to some of our cool discoveries, like the river that's now a linear park—Jardin del Turia Gardens. So, how did the river Turia become a beautiful, seven-kilometre-long park? It all happened because of a flood, a river diverted, a community coming together to protect their beloved Valencia, and government officials willing to change their minds about building a highway from Madrid to Valencia. This was in favour of gardens created for locals and tourists to bike, walk, relax, play football, sip wine or coffee, and appreciate the eighteen bridges that spanned the gardens. A great deal of money was invested to move—yes, *move*—the river.

The Jardin del Turia is also home to the City of Arts and Science, a place many folks strongly suggested we visit. We decided to do so mid-week. Tickets purchased, we arrived at our first stop, the Oceanografic, just in time for opening. I realise that some folks take issue with animals being captive in such places… I respect that. However, from our perspective, this was an amazing place to visit. We were in awe of the beauty of the animals and their habitats, carefully and thoughtfully designed buildings, pools, aviaries… all created to maximize visitors' ability to appreciate the viewing while respecting the needs of its inhabitants. visibility, interaction where appropriate, and immense beauty to behold. If you are having a bad day, I would encourage you to walk around and take in these amazing creations. I guarantee you would quickly find yourself smiling, laughing, and simply in awe.

Next step... follow up your Oceanografic adventure with a visit to the Hemisfèric. We chose to see the Blue Ocean, and once more, we were in awe. This IMAX Cinema boasts a digital 3D screen measuring about twenty-two by eleven metres. It was huge! The chairs were in a semi-lying position, enabling the guests to view the most spectacular under and above-water life imaginable. To be sure, the message of preserving our oceans came across loud and clear! The last stop in our visit to the Ciudad de las Artes y las Ciencias was the Arts and Science Centre. While we all enjoyed the exhibits as adults, we couldn't help thinking how much our grandchildren would have been enthralled by the endless hands-on activities offered.

By this time, we were exhausted and ready to head back to Cabanyal for dinner at another of our favourite eateries, La Princesa Restaurante. Once more, the food was amazing, and we thoroughly enjoyed a great conversation about the joys and wonders we had just experienced, and of course, the ever-present challenge of ordering food in an area where English is little understood. The confusion was such that we ended up paying for four desserts rather than two, five sangrias (which were amazing) rather than three, and devoured a delicious dish of venison cheeks we didn't order. We also turned away two more plates of food not requested. The overcharges on the bill weren't noticed until later; to their credit, when our friends approached La Princesa the next day. They immediately righted the mistake and all was well.

A walking tour of Old Town on Thursday was capped with a trip to the Valencia Central Market, where our friends purchased what was reputed to be the best olive oil in Spain (recommended by our paella chefs). Following another superb gastronomical treat, three of us climbed the 207 steps of the Miguelete Bell Tower of Valencia's Cathedral and were rewarded with a spectacular view of the city—and the 4 p.m. chime of the bells directly above our heads! Two euros well spent.

One thing you need to know about our friends: music is a shared passion. We are not just music observers, but performers, composers, music teachers, orchestra members, pianists extraordinaire, and vocalists. Needless to say, when we learned that renowned oboe player Francois Leleux was performing with the Valencia Orchestra under the direction of conductor and artistic director Alexander Liebreich, purchasing tickets was a must. The concert was inspiring, uplifting, and memorable. The Auditori seats 1,490 spectators and was truly spectacular. It was in the same area as La Ciutat de les Arts i les Ciències.

Our friends left at the end of the week to explore more of Spain, but in that short week, we created more wonderful memories to add to our many adventures together. There is no doubt how difficult it was to be away from family and friends as we sojourned in Europe, making us all the more thankful for the time to share our journey with them. They will always be part of our story.

CHAPTER 20

Life is not measured by the number of breaths we take, but by the moments that take our breath away.

—Maya Angelou

Córdoba was a place we didn't have time to explore; however, it was an added bonus to visit another Spanish city, noted to be one of Andalucía's most fascinating cities, home to four UNESCO Heritage Sites. For our one night in Cordova, we stayed at the Hotel Centre, a lovely hotel with excellent access to the older part of town. We did have time mid-afternoon through the evening to explore Old Town and browse the lovely stores and take in the delightful wares produced by local artisans. One such place sold the most beautiful silk scarves, a little above my price range (OK, a lot above my price range), but my husband did buy me a beautiful silver rose scarf magnet. Flowers, I learned, are very important to the Spanish people, often symbolising various emotions. The rose speaks of everlasting love—what a fitting gift! I often wondered how the ladies in Spain kept their scarves so neatly in place without damaging the delicate silk most were made from. Their secret? Magnets rather than pins! Brilliant.

I'm into views... rooftop views over cities or views from the top of cliffs looking over an ocean or the Mediterranean Sea. Then, there are balcony views over the goings-on of life on the sidewalks and streets below. We've marvelled at the views from the top of the Duomo in Florence, or the Miguelete Bell Tower in Valencia, and will never forget standing on Mars Hill, overlooking the impressive city of Athens. Views give you a different perspective—they remind you to take a step back and see the bigger picture.

In April, we took a ten-day visit to the Algarve. For this visit, we stayed in Carvoeiro, a five-minute drive to Lagoa, where our family was staying. We had discovered Carvoeiro while living in Albufeira and had found it such a delightful place. Now, after staying there for ten days, we absolutely loved it. There's just something about the town and its natural beauty. Of course, the views over the Atlantic were breathtaking, the cafés and restaurants plentiful, and while most servers were Portuguese their mastery of the English language really helped when our Portuguese skills amounted to *bom dia* and *obrigada*!

The town had a lovely combination of new and old structures, many restored to reflect Portuguese heritage. We also found the people to be warm and welcoming, as was fairly common everywhere in Portugal. For us, Carvoeiro was a perfect, central location for day trips to other amazing beaches, towns, and cities, like Lagos or Portimão. It also offered incredible hiking along clifftops. Just to give you a glimpse of what I mean, this was the view just across the street from our vacation rental.

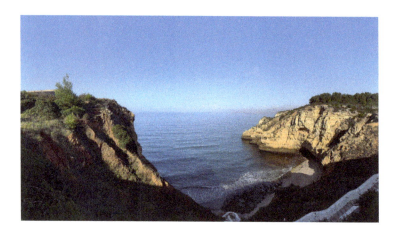

Carvoeiro

The reason for the visit back to Portugal? A family reunion. Our family had been spread all over the globe for some time, so this was a treasured time to be together—time for European Uncle and Auntie to finally meet their new niece, and for our son's children to meet their Canadian cousin for the first time. It was love at first sight. There's nothing like relaxing on a beautiful Algarve beach, sun shining, water sparkling, while the grandkids and Papa try to build a sandcastle, laughter all around... basking in the simple joys of life. As for the older kids? Uncle Jordan and I busied ourselves trying to get a game of beach volleyball going—not an easy task when the sport was a totally new experience for them. Still, we laughed, lunged, and clumsily faltered when trying to go for a setup... not graceful, but certainly a great time.

For me personally, being with family can provide a fresh perspective. It reminds me I'm not alone in the world, and that the children my husband and I raised have grown into adults who both reflect the values we instilled in them and have acquired wisdom beyond anything we, as parents, passed on to them.

Then there are the grandchildren… oh my! Seeing your offspring and their spouses raise their own children is the moment you can step back and know the future is in good hands—a beautiful thing.

For those ten days in April, we had our emotional tanks refilled, creating new memories with our children, their spouses, and all seven grandkids. To say that this time with our family was a healing balm to my mental and emotional health would be an understatement. I remember sitting outside by the pool at the home our son and his family were renting. As I often did during our time away, I found myself focusing on the way the future would be greatly impacted by my husband's health. The tears were once again flowing. How, in the midst of such joy and memory-making, could this fear of impending doom hit again? It happens! Just then, my son came to check on me. I'm not great at hiding my emotions—especially where my kids are concerned. They can see right through me. The words Nathan spoke—so filled with love, compassion, empathy, hope, and support—were exactly what I needed. I wasn't alone, nor would I ever be. The conversation ended with a tight, warm, assuring hug that only a son can give his mum. It was later that same day when my daughter expressed her own support, echoing what her brother had said, punctuated with another warm, loving, assuring hug. What a gift.

Vistas, new perspectives, memory-making… we have had a lifetime of such treasures. While the family was together in Portugal, we spent time exploring some of the wonderful, sandy beaches previously introduced to us by our explorer daughter-in-law. We also revisited some other special places, one being Monchique. Besides the desire to show it off to our daughter and family, we wanted to bring them to the very place where, only a couple of months earlier, Shannon and Jordan had video called to share the exciting news that we would once again welcome a little blessing to the family. Such joy! (Zachary was born a couple of months following our return from Europe.) The wonders of technology allowed our whole family to celebrate the joyous news together.

We enjoyed many hours together playing games—Monopoly, Settlers of Catan, and Uno (all six versions of it). And of course, the challenge was on to see if the older kids could beat Gramma at Wordle! In case you're wondering, I was outsmarted by my grandkids more times than I care to mention. Evenings would often find the kids gathered around Papa in front of the fire as he read them whatever story they chose… usually Abby's choice, since she was the youngest. Speaking of views—how lovely is the view of your grandkids playing together?

There have been other places we've visited whose views were so impressive that, when recalled, could transport me to that moment in time. The place that immediately comes to mind is Santorini, one of the Greek Islands. We visited there in 2013 with some friends, the same ones who came to Valencia. Incredibly beautiful. Now, we are really fortunate that two of the friends we travel with love to design the actual trip and research the many sights and wonders one shouldn't miss. On this Greek island holiday, Mr. W. chose and booked all our accommodations. Each location—Athens, Samos, Mykonos, Naxos, Santorini, and Nafplio—was spectacular, but when we arrived at our cave house in Santorini and walked out to our private balcony, the view took our breath away. The Mediterranean had never looked so majestic, and we could sit on our large balcony and take it all in. All those pictures of Greece featured in travel magazines didn't do it justice. On top of the amazing view, each morning, the Airbnb hostess delivered fresh bread for breakfast. It doesn't get much better than that. A close second was the view from our private balcony in Naxos, overlooking the same sea.

We experienced another amazing view just a couple of weeks

before returning to Canada. It was early in the day when we arrived at the hotel. We opened the curtains of our room only to be awestruck by the view from our hotel balcony. This is what we would feast our eyes on for the next six mornings!

Can you recall a memory of a special childhood vacation that never seems to fade over the passing years? Imagine something with me. I'm standing on a hotel balcony, the warm breeze gently touching my skin, soft music dancing all around, the murmurs of people basking in the Mediterranean sun mixing with the gentle ebb and flow of the sea. My mind flashes back to an almost twelve-year-old pre-teen experiencing Ibiza for the very first time. The warmth, the hum of families playing in the pool, the sky bluer than I'd ever seen, and the possibilities of new adventures ahead.

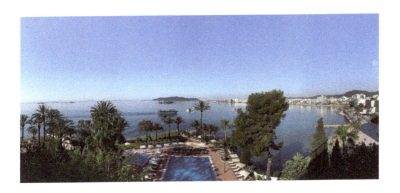

Ibiza

They say that memories exaggerate things, but Ibiza was every bit as beautiful as I remembered. Fifty-three years later, back again, I could close my eyes and relive those delicious memories like it was yesterday.

When laying out our schedule for Europe, Ibiza had not been on the list. Bilbao and San Sebastian were strong contenders; however, after a few long days of driving between Portugal and Spain, we decided to find something closer to our place in Valencia. It was only then that Ibiza came into the picture. Travel there involved a five-minute drive to the ferry in Valencia, an overnight ferry to Ibiza, and another ten-minute drive to our hotel. Perfect!

For six days, we lazed by the pool, read and listened to audiobooks, walked the promenade, explored Dalt Vila (Old Town) ate delicious meals, drank excellent Spanish wines, and treated ourselves to a three-hour sunset cruise on a thirty-five-foot sailboat while enjoying a lovely charcuterie served with Cava. That's it. No tight schedule, no rushing, just relaxation.

At one point, my husband asked, "So, what have you been thinking about while sitting out here?"

"Nothing, absolutely nothing" was my immediate response.

Now, if you know me, you'll know that's a totally uncharacteristic reality for my mind...for it to be so at peace, so quiet, so *present* is a rare happening. Not until the question was posed did I fully realise how completely relaxed and free of concern I actually was. Ibiza has a reputation for being a party island. That's true, to a certain extent, but not where we were. The rowdiest noisemakers were the birds... and their song was most welcome. We needed that downtime and our six-hour overnight ferry ride from Valencia to Ibiza had transported us to the perfect retreat.

I thought I would be inspired to do some writing, to dream of the future, but no... all I wanted to do was take in the peace, tranquillity, and beauty around us.

That wouldn't be our final experience with amazing views on the adventure.

Madrid... what an amazing city! Two days was not enough to really get to know a place, but certainly enough to leave an impression. The architecture was incredible—the buildings, the balconies, and the most spectacular statues everywhere we looked. We stayed at the Iberostar, which provided some of the best customer service we've ever experienced. From the hotel, we walked, and walked, and absorbed all that is Madrid.

On the first day, we just wandered, coming first to the Plaza Mayor, then took in the San Miguel Market, which offered the most amazing display of tapas I have ever seen! Next, we headed to Almudena Cathedral and were awed by its majesty. One aspect I really appreciated was the colour of the ceilings and stained-glass windows—beautiful. Fun fact: Real Madrid CF won the UEFA Champions League final the day before we arrived. The following day, they offered the trophy to the Virgin of Almudena, along with a beautiful bouquet of flowers. On our visit, I climbed to the platform where the flowers had been laid—a part of Madrid's history.

Day two was a very different experience, though still amazing. We ended the day at the Museo Del Prado. If you have time for only one museum, this is the one. The art is exquisite, including the many statues throughout. We were even treated to a young woman playing classical piano as we wandered the many rooms. A multi-sensory delight.

As terrific as the Prado was, the majority of our second day was spent strolling around one of the most peaceful, beautiful parks I have encountered, Parque del Retiro. If someone were just dropped into El Retiro, they would never guess they were in the middle of a city hosting a population of about 6.7 million people! There was so much to appreciate about this UNESCO World Heritage Site: a lovely lake with row boats, over 128 hectares of green space, 15,000 trees, the colourful and fragrant La Rosaleda Garden (with over 4,000 roses), countless majestic statues that told much of the history of Madrid. Perhaps the most spectacular feature of the park was the Palacio de Cristal ("Glass Palace"), dating back to 1887. The sun beaming through the windows created a surreal experience as we walked through this building constructed of glass and iron, The name Parque del Retiro means "Pleasant Retreat Park," a perfect description of the oasis for gaining perspective and creating a memorable experience during our final days in Europe.

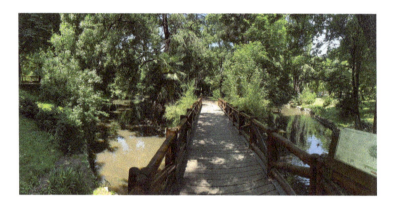

Parque de El Retiro

What is it about views that provide such an opportunity for reflection and refreshment for overwhelmed souls? For paving the way to a changed perspective? Perhaps it's simply the way such vistas cause us to slow down, stop, take in our surroundings, marvel at what we see, bracket whatever is happening in our day-to-day lives, and whisper a prayer of thanksgiving to the Creator for what has unfolded before our eyes.

CHAPTER 21

There is no mile as long the final one that leads back home.
—Katherine Marsh

At the writing of this short chapter, we were sitting in the airport lounge in Vancouver, ready to embark on the final leg of our journey home. Over the past few hours, we had flown from Madrid to Toronto, then on to Vancouver. In less than an hour, we would board the plane for the short one-hour flight to Kelowna, back home.

Four weeks previous we had made a major decision. Due to some of the challenges presented in Valencia, combined with my husband's growing desire to get back to Canada and his medical team, we decided to return home four weeks earlier than we had originally planned. It was a difficult decision, but when it came to my husband's health, it was a no-brainer.

Travelling to Europe and living abroad for this length of time had been no easy task for someone with end-stage renal failure, but Rob had done it. His optimism, endurance, and sense of adventure provided the impetus to keep going. But we both knew the decision was a wise one—certainly not indicative of any kind of failure. We were both at peace with it. We were also grateful for our travel agent back in Canada, who took care of our flight changes home from Madrid to Kelowna, transfers, and our overnight hotel on the way home.

It truly had been an amazing seven-month journey, an unforgettable life experience that will take some time to fully process… time to reflect on the ups, downs, joys, tears, surprises, memories, and life lessons (which still come along no matter your age). I have always believed travel opens our eyes to a fantastic world that changes us forever.

For now, we look forward to arriving at the Kelowna airport into the open arms of our daughter and granddaughter. Such joy awaits!

CHAPTER 22

Travel isn't always pretty. It isn't always comfortable. Sometimes it hurts. It even breaks your heart. But that's OK. The journey changes you; it should change you. It leaves marks on your memory, on your consciousness, on your heart, and on your body. You take something with you. Hopefully, you leave something good behind.

—Anthony Bourdain

We had been home for just over a week. People kept asking how it felt to be back home. To be honest, I wasn't quite sure how to answer, and still struggle with it. Yes, it was amazing to be back with family and friends, and yes, it was wonderful to be back in our own home. But we missed Europe. There was a sense of longing that settled in—a longing to go back to places that, for a time, had been our second home.

I went for my first bike ride a week after arriving home, on what I affectionately call my "girly-bike" (a baby blue cruiser). Riding along a close-by linear park, Mission Creek, it felt good to take in familiar sights, sounds and smells once again. In the afternoon, beach chairs slung on our backs, my husband and I took the short walk to the Okanagan Lake and breathed in the beauty that was before us. Back home, we sat on the deck with a glass of wine and olives, reliving the many afternoon wine-sipping breaks we had enjoyed in Portugal and Spain. It was wonderful to bask in our gratitude for the many wonderful experiences of the past seven months.

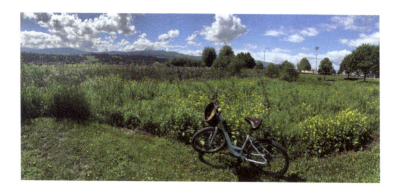

That was our second week at home. Week one had not been so peaceful and tranquil. One of the many lessons we learned while travelling was that the first week in a new location is always wrought with a sense of total upheaval. Arriving back in Kelowna felt somewhat the same. While it was familiar, it wasn't yet *home* again. Things had changed. New buildings had been erected, prices of food and gas had skyrocketed, our grocery store no longer sold our favourite Sunday morning scones, our condo was a shell, void of personal items, and pneumonia arrived home from Europe with my husband, resulting in two days of emergency room visits in a hospital greatly suffering the effects of extremely low staffing (fallout from the pandemic). It felt like we had simply moved to the next location on our journey.

Eventually, we did settle in. In those settling-in days, I sat in my home office or on the deck, writing or preparing for fall teaching, looking out at blue skies and vibrant green trees.

Our walls once again housed the smiling pictures of our adored kids and grandkids, updated from our travels. Familiar books, like old friends, once again lined the shelves, and a cup of hot coffee accompanied my morning quietness.

It was good to be home, truly home. Our time with family and friends was richer than ever, our appreciation of where we lived had grown, and our gratitude for my husband's amazing medical team was even stronger than before we had left for Europe.

But there was a change, I could feel it. In me. I couldn't explain it, but was aware of it and looked forward to digging deeper and reflecting on how Europe had taken root in my soul.

During the third week home, I was engaged in three days of strategic planning with our college business department. Excitement to reconnect with colleagues was quickly replaced with a sense of being an outsider. I'm not sure how else to describe how I felt. It had been ten months since the start of my leave, but before that, our offices on campus had been vacated due to the pandemic. December 2019 through the end of March 2020 found me at home on medical leave, recovering from a knee replacement; a week after my gradual return to work, we were all sent home to teach online because of COVID-19. It wasn't until the Fall of 2021 that face-to-face classes fully resumed—just when I had started my study leave.

In an encouraging conversation with a colleague I greatly respect, he let me know he had also experienced this outsider feeling following each of the three extended study leaves he had taken. Sitting in those meetings was almost like a time warp. Conversations were the same, problems needing to be addressed hadn't changed much. The *welcome homes* I had expected were few and far between. In fact, many of the faculty didn't even realise I had been gone—such was the reality of teaching when weeks and months would go by without professors even seeing one another, save passing in the halls between classes. For most, life in our beautiful city, working in a highly respected college, focusing on the challenges at hand, continued as per usual... but not for me.

I wanted to stand up and shout, "Listen, people, there's a big, exciting world out there and we need to prepare our students for a future that is full of opportunity and never-before-experienced challenges. Our main focus may be to serve our community, but our community is no longer confined to local boundaries. It is already—and will continue to be—part of a global community. That's where our mindset needs to go! We need to pave the way, lead by example, and be agents of change in our strategic planning and in the classrooms. Every conversation with students should leave them challenged to move beyond their current worldview to that of a global citizen, where conversations of diversity, equity, and inclusion no longer need to happen because they are part of our DNA." But I couldn't. It wasn't the time or the place. But someday, sometime…

In one-on-one conversations with a few like-minded colleagues, we share our eagerness to be part of something great, to think of practical, tangible ways to effect change and to adjust the direction of the big ship that is a fitting metaphor for educational institutions. For me, a person of action, change isn't happening quickly enough and seems to be hampered by the many layers of bureaucracy so common in the education industry. I greatly appreciate the efforts and initiative of our business department leadership team, but even their hands are tied when it comes to moving forward in a timely manner.

I'm not sure how long I will be part of the world of formal education, but for now, there are approximately 180 students I have the honour and responsibility to teach each semester. I get excited about the potential conversations that will emerge from young, eager minds whose common desire is to leave their mark on the world, making it a better place than it was when it was passed on to them. I look forward to embracing the many different cultures of the people sitting at their desks or on the screen in front of me, learning from them, and providing a safe environment where their differences can be discussed and tough issues addressed. I want to foster conversations among my students, domestic and international, in the context of what we study regarding leadership, human resources, and organisational behaviour. I look forward to sharing my experience from our time abroad, the joys and challenges, the barriers and breakthroughs—and, most of all, the opportunity *they* have to live and work anywhere they choose.

Travel changes a person... it's inevitable. We don't always know how, but it does. You bring a bit of each place you visit home with you and leave a part of yourself in each place you have sojourned. Travel feeds and deepens your curiosity, grows your appreciation and respect for other cultures and people, broadens your palate for new tastes in foods, forces you to reflect on why you do the things you do, and nourishes a deep love for life. It's addictive! Travel changes how you view the life you've lived and have yet to live. It challenges your *why*. The lens through which you see the world changes. I sincerely hope it has changed me... how could it not?

CHAPTER 23, EPILOGUE

Gratitude was never meant to be an excuse for giving up on the obstacles God has put before you. Some of the most magical things He can bring us require faith and a lot of planning.

—Shannon L. Alder

I don't know if you are a fan of makeover TV shows. From house rebuilds, redecorating, or restorations to personal makeovers involving diet, professional life, personal appearance, relationships, finances... name any area of life, and you can be guaranteed a makeover TV show has been created to focus on it. There's something about the opportunity for a re-do that is appealing to us humans, no matter how satisfied we are with life.

While on this journey, my husband and I know we didn't do everything right. But that's OK. Often, we simply didn't know the questions to ask or the processes to follow. At times, we made decisions based on assumptions, while at other times, decisions were made for us. We often talk about what a re-do might look like for our time living and researching abroad. In other words, if we again planned such a trip, be it for research, to write a book, or combine retirement from full-time work with freelance work, what might that look like? How would our experience inform the why, what, where, when, and how of such a trip? Let me try to articulate what that might look like based on a checklist of questions we had asked and answered before heading out the first time.

1. **Why do you want to do this?** What's your impetus? What's your purpose? Over the course of my extended study leave, I was often asked why I chose to live in Europe while most of the research and interviews were conducted virtually. I didn't need to leave the comfort of my home in Canada to complete the project. But for me, the experience of living a remote lifestyle was an important part of the research. Remember, I'm the person who got yelled at by guards for touching Giorgio Vasari's breathtaking frescoes while touring the Duomo di Firenze. The committee responsible for approving my study plan easily grasped the research element of my study leave as the rationale for why I was focusing my study on leadership in hybrid and remote teams. However, the lived experience aspect of my proposal was not as clear to them, but the following helped them understand:

    - The growth of remote work is allowing individuals to be location-independent. I wanted to experience first-hand what that looked like.

    - I wanted to experience the challenges (and joys) faced by remote workers (at the time of writing the proposal I didn't realise these would include major medical issues).

    - Many individuals in the younger Baby Boomer generation (of which I am one) are not ready to retire but do not want to remain in a nine-to-five job for the final years of their working lives. Freedom to travel and work is more attractive, and long for as this generation seeks out more flexible work arrangements. I wanted to experience what that looked like.

- Living in an area is the best way to understand the culture. Culture greatly influences people's views of work. I wanted to get a sense of that culture in various locations.

As you can see, my *why* spoke to both professional and personal reasons. you will need to determine this for yourself. Further consideration will lead you to determine if your *why* is about exploration or gaining new perspectives. Might it be to mark or celebrate a life transition, like reaching an age milestone, an empty nest, or perhaps retirement? Or might it be more about a personal life transition, perhaps following a traumatic event or loss? Perhaps it is a trip of personal discovery. It may even be as simple as you being worn out and needing a break. Only you will be able to articulate the *why* behind your decision to embark on an adventure. However, your *why* will inform and impact every subsequent decision you make.

2. **What do you want to do?** Your *why* is going to help answer this question. I did not want to live in the midst of vacationers—or even expatriates. I wanted to see and experience the culture as lived by those who called the area home. That meant hotel stays were out (along with the expense!). I wanted to live as the locals lived, whatever that meant. I remember being a youngster growing up in Bangor, heading to the local market twice a week with my Mum to get fresh fruits and vegetables, then making

a stop at Johnny's Meats to pick up the best sausages ever. Less frequent visits just wouldn't suffice, as our fridge, like most in Europe, couldn't hold anymore. I wanted to relive that memory as an adult. In some way, I wanted to live a simpler life and experience the ups and downs that accompany that choice. I wanted to learn what it would be like to experience work, life, and leisure in such a context.

3. **Where do you want to go?** If you need inspiration as to *where* you want to go, there is no end to the amazing websites, books, and blogs full of ideas, experiences, and suggestions to get your planning juices flowing. I remember a couple of books that certainly got me thinking about different locations:: *The Alchemist* by Paulo Coelho and *Wild* by Cheryl Strayed, to name two. I recently found a website that listed "The 100 Greatest Travel Books of All Time." However, don't lose sight of your *why* and *what*. Just because it's possible to go to a certain location doesn't mean it's the right location for you. At the start of our planning journey, my husband and I created a checklist of what we would look for in potential locations in which to live. Over the planning time, the checklist needed to be adjusted and adapted to our needs—especially those related to my husband's medical condition. Some items were very specific, others more vague. The locations we selected need to:

- Be in close proximity to our son and family, at some point

- Have a mild, temperate climate so we didn't have to pack clothes for the Canadian type of winter

- Be close to the sea or ocean—preferably within walking distance

- Have good public transportation so we wouldn't need to rent a car
- Be a location that would allow for day or weekend trips exploring the region
- Have character and history (easy to find in Europe)
- Offer a strong Internet connection
- Have co-working spaces for alternate *work-from* locations
- Allow us to get by with English as our only language
- Have accessibility to nephrology support in hospitals and medical labs
- Be locations where the pharmaceutical company would deliver my husband's medical supplies

Fortunately, the possibilities were great and varied. Our final selections each met most of the criteria. In Albufeira, we did need a car, since public transit between places wasn't as accessible—an easy problem to solve (albeit hard on the budget). The language barrier in Valencia was the greatest criterion not met; it was, however, a huge lesson learned for us.

4. **When can you go?** For me, the *when* was clear. Professionally, I knew that after a certain number of years at the college, I would qualify for an extended study leave. But equally important was the timing when my husband could accompany me. With his recent retirement, the timing worked perfectly. But then we needed to consider the reality of his health. The medical team had to contribute to this decision. For you, there will be other things to consider as far as timing is concerned, as unique to you as

the trip you take will be. *When* is really a big-picture decision, because the rest of life doesn't pause just because we have a desire to engage in extended travel. None of us live in isolation, so consider your community and how it will be impacted. Don't rush through this. In the excitement of the potential journey, it is easy to ignore how others may be impacted by your decision, so speak with family, friends, work colleagues, volunteer groups, medical advisors, and whomever else may be in your circle.

5. **How can you make it happen?** This is an exciting one… especially if you are a planner. This is the area where barriers and obstacles can often raise their heads, and doubt can set in. *Believe me, I know!* But don't be discouraged, there is just about always a way through—or around—any challenge.

    As you can imagine, medical issues were a big one for us. The obstacles seemed to increase at every turn. But, as you have read, with the help and support of an amazing medical team, family, and friends, each obstacle was crushed. A friend often reminds us that a medical condition shouldn't define you. For us, travel looks a lot different than it used to, but it is still an important part of our lives from which we derive joy.

    For many, finances will be another hurdle that may threaten to squash plans. Travel expenses will be unique to your situation, so once a travel decision is made, a focus on pre-trip savings is critical. Like us, you may find medical conditions require additional travel insurance; BCAA was the only provider we could find that offered what we needed. A bonus came when a friend recommended a colleague interested in renting our home for the duration of our trip—the rental income covered our accommodations in Europe.

The cost of living in a location also plays a key factor in finances. We knew the cost of living in both Portugal and Spain was lower than in Canada so that obviously influenced our location choices.

With this knowledge in hand, we created a budget that included all the obvious expenses, as well as extra spending for exploring the beauty and surprises offered in both countries. My husband kept careful records of how each dollar was spent, and I'm pleased to say we didn't miss out on anything.

Other *hows* need to be addressed, such as how to work from other locations. You may be breaking new ground in your organisation, but it's well worth the effort—especially if it means paving the way for others. The growth in remote, hybrid, and work-from-anywhere arrangements makes such travel adventures more possible.

However, it is important to work with your organisation (if not already a remote worker) to ensure both data security and tax implications have been considered. When discussing tax implications, your human resources department should be able to advise—and if this is a new area for them, a quick search on platforms such as LinkedIn will connect you with appropriate experts.

All things considered, our trip turned out better than we could ever have imagined. However, there are four things we learned and would incorporate into our do-over...

1. The most important element in communication is language, so beginning to learn the language ahead of time is important.
2. Moving from observing and experiencing a culture to being part of it takes time—more than four months.

3. When you commit to a longer timeframe, it would be valuable to first reach out to an expatriate community, then branch out to the local community.

4. You must put aside any assumptions and judgments you have about a culture, and be open to learning and appreciating the history behind what may be some of the craziest traditions you have ever seen!

Two questions remain: would we do it again if the opportunity presented itself? And would we recommend this experience to others? The answer to both is *without a doubt, yes*! I would also add that my husband and I take "in sickness and in health" seriously. Never let health issues be a barrier to experiencing some of the greatest adventures life has to offer.

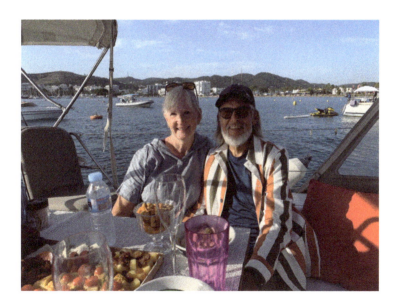

Heading out on a sunset sail, Ibiza

Don't cry because it's over, smile because it happened.
—Dr. Seuss

APPENDIX A: THE RESEARCH

For those readers interested in learning more about my research, I've written a chapter just for you. If you are interested in reading my published papers regarding the research, all are available through my website. https://www.samisremote.com/

It is a capital mistake to theorise before you have all the evidence. It biases the judgement.

—"Sherlock Holmes" in the novel
A Study in Scarlet by Arthur Conan Doyle (1887)

As you know by now, I am a business professor, as well as a coach and trainer who focuses on supporting leaders and teams in flexible working contexts. I have appreciated the privilege of adopting a form of work from anywhere for most of my professional life. In my early career, my employers fully supported me working in the office or from home—whatever I needed. I have enjoyed colocated offices as well as a home office, teaching amazing students in face-to-face classroom settings as well as fully online, and working from amazing coffee shops in North America and Europe—all the while, ensuring the strong work ethic I was raised with. I fully embrace the advice offered by Richard Branson: "If somebody offers you an amazing opportunity but you are not sure you can do it, say yes—then learn how to do it later!"

That day back in October 2019 when I received the approval for my research, it took quite a while to peel me off the roof—and needless to say, my eyes glistened with tears of joy. What this meant was that for a full year, I would be able to focus on an area I was and continue to be very passionate about. The initial research, conducted with our son Nathan, focused on competencies for success as remote workers. That initial experience introduced me to so many amazing people both in North America and Europe.

I have always felt strongly about the role of leadership. I take it very seriously and highly respect those who take the posture of a reluctant leader. Psychologist Dan B. Allender authored a book back in 2011 entitled *Leading with a Limp: Take Full Advantage of Your Most Powerful Weakness*.[7] Early in 2020, many leaders began to realise the way they had always done leadership no longer worked. They found themselves *leading with a limp*. And I greatly admired them. They had to hit the ground running, limp and all. I wanted to learn from, such leaders, and then share what I had learned with the myriad individuals out there leading teams and organizations in an era of continual change.

Have you ever been on your way to an appointment—perhaps with a client or for a social event—and were met with unexpected construction, causing you to be unfashionably late? Or perhaps you were set to make a presentation, only to discover the Internet gremlins had done their worst causing the connection

---

[7] Dan B. Allender, *Leading with a Limp: Take Full Advantage of Your Most Powerful Weakness*," (Waterbrook, 2011).

to be less than adequate? I have, and it was not a pretty sight! Adjustments, re-arrangements, rescheduling, and great apologies were made before things got back on track. Things happen—things outside our control—that call for change. It takes time to get our head into a new arrangement, to get over the frustration of the disruption, to recalibrate, and to settle on what appears to be a *less-than* outcome. But is it always?

Some changes are totally beyond our control. When I began my research, most organisations were being forced to make a change to their standard operating procedures. Life in the office as we had known it was no more—but not because we chose it... the decision had been made for us. In a matter of days—even hours—organisations had to do a whirlwind pivot. No time for preparation, no time for analysis, no time for decision-making—the move was pretty much instantaneous. Being thrown into the deep end means you either sink or swim. Sadly, we've witnessed both.

Some may think the outcome is a less-than-result. However, I beg to differ. To be sure, a disequilibrium has been created in which we have to live, but until it happened, many organisations, or employees, would not have considered the opportunities provided by a work-from-anywhere or hybrid concept of working.

Many organisations made the switch with reasonable success, but others were devastated and are still transitioning. We are seeing growth in a hybrid option for work. Working from anywhere has become a concept organisations are getting their collective heads around as both employers and employees witness the benefits of moving away from traditional co-located workforces. The narrative around remote work has changed—and continues to.

My intent as I embarked on my research was not to focus on the benefits to all involved with working from anywhere but rather to put it in the context of change. To bring attention to how we, as leaders of people, had been handed a mulligan, a do-over. We had an opportunity to do business differently, to adapt rather than mourn the loss of how things used to be; to take advantage of an unplanned change and create the next phase of how we work, where we work, when we work, and what work we do. And it all had to focus on the people.

Fast forward to today, and we see a world that has changed in ways none of us could ever have imagined. Many are still waving the flag for employees to return full-time *to the office*, others have transitioned from working from home to being remote workers who can work from anywhere, and others are still transitioning to a hybrid way of working. I'm not saying any of this was or is easy... far from it. Leaders are called to be pioneers in this journey of discovery and transition, and to practise adaptive leadership. As Heifetz, Grashow, and Linsky say, "To practise adaptive leadership, you have to help people navigate through a period of disturbance as they sift through what is essential and what is expendable, and as they experiment with solutions to the adaptive challenges at hand"[8].

It took many months to figure out what I wanted to research and then put a proposal together that would make sense from an academic and industry perspective. I knew I wanted to once again integrate evidence-based research with stories and examples from industry. I wanted to hear the stories of how individuals had transitioned from co-located work to working from home to working from anywhere—or to hybrid work. I wanted to learn what they found to be effective and what did not work. I also wanted to learn (and share) the reasons behind what worked, and what didn't, in leading work-from-anywhere

---

8 R. Heifetz, A. Grashow, and M. Linsky, *The Practice of Adaptive Leadership: Tools and Tactics for Changing Your Organization and the World* (Harvard Business Review Press, 2009).

teams. In hearing the stories, I wanted to encourage those I interviewed to join me on the balcony, to look back over the journeys they had taken, and perhaps even recognise where they may have taken a wrong turn.

The proposal preparation process was challenging, to say the least. I am an impatient person. Multi-tasking comes easy and being in the midst of the action is stimulating for me. My mind works fast. I receive information and quickly sort through it to get to a resolution. Making decisions is easy. However, through the school of hard knocks, I have learned that impatience, action, quick assimilation of information, multi-tasking, and fast decision-making are not always good things. In fact, they're rarely good things when, as leaders, we are faced with making decisions that impact those we are called to serve and support. I soon learned to appreciate the rigour involved in putting together a detailed research proposal, that would enable me to stand before our research and ethics board and support the validity of my proposal.

Many people have heard of the concept of a "balcony view." It refers to the mental (or physical) action of stepping back and gaining perspective. I first heard about it shortly after visiting the Cathedral of Santa Maria del Fiore, the Duomo, in Florence. We had spent a few days visiting places like the Galleria Dell' Accademia and were moved by Michel Angelo's David, an impressive seventeen-foot statue of detailed strength and beauty. We leisurely walked through the Uffizi Gallery, awed by magnificent paintings by artists like Raphael, Botticelli, and da Vinci. And of course, we delighted in the many cafés with their delicious pastries and memorable coffee.

After walking many miles, our final adventure was to climb the 463 steps to the top of the Duomo. The staircase quickly narrowed to a spiral climb—suffocating for a claustrophobic! However, once we broke into the warmth of the afternoon sun, we were rewarded with the most magnificent view... Florence from 114 metres above! We could trace the path of our explorations, see each location in relation to the others, and even notice places we didn't realise existed. I think you get where I'm going with this.

Let me get a little academic here: Heifetz, Grashow, and Linsky added to the balcony view concept by referring to the action of *"moving from the dance floor to the balcony."* We love the dance floor. We love being at the heart of the action, enjoying the energy of everyone dancing to the same beat. It's difficult to pull ourselves away, to step up to the balcony and be an observer rather than a participant. But as leaders, we must, and sometimes we need to be invited to do so.

But what are we doing on the balcony? Heifetz and his co-authors suggest three activities in which we need to engage: observe, interpret, and intervene.

If you were to ask me or one of my friends what we saw from the top of the Duomo, we would each have described something different—all correct, but different. This is an important part of observing. We look at things through the lens of our personal experience and bias, so when on the balcony, our view or perspective is broadened to include a view of the everyday workings of our team or organisation. The authors encourage leaders to then move into the practice of interpreting what they have observed. Once more, we need to acknowledge the fact that we interpret our observations differently than our colleagues, and check our assumptions. In our human desire to get to solutions, we may rush through this interpreting stage. Taking time to consider, ponder, and reflect will enhance our accuracy in deciphering what our senses take in. This pause will greatly impact the interventions or actions we undertake.

What exactly am I trying to get across here? As I planned to engage in conversation with 150-plus individuals through this research, I wanted to see how our conversations might move through their observations of remote and hybrid leadership to their interpretations of what it meant, and finally to learn how they intervene in order to continue applying and adapting what they learn.

As I embarked on my project, I was excited to learn, relearn, have my opinions challenged, and contribute my findings to the many individuals, teams, and organisations facing challenging and exciting transitions in how and where work gets done. My earlier research, focused on remote workers. This led to a research project with Ian MacRae looking at the personality traits of remote workers.[9] Looking back, never would we have predicted the importance of our research for a time of such global disruption.

What was next? Where would my focus land? The overarching question I sought to find answers to was "What does it take to lead successfully in a work-from-anywhere context, ensuring proximity equity?" I wanted to hear stories from both leaders and team members regarding how they experienced proximity equity, especially when discussing access to resources (support, training, data, promotions, collaboration, and so on.). Conversely, there is much to be learned from individuals who fall victim to proximity bias—meaning, those who are overlooked for promotions, excluded from face-to-face events and social activities, or whose access to necessary resources is otherwise limited due to their geographical locations. Their stories also needed to be heard. Many of the interviewees were still in the early stages of new working contexts, while others had been experiencing hybrid

---

9   Ian MacRae and Roberta Sawatzky, "Remote Working: Personality and Performance Research Results" Research Gate (2020). https://www.academia.edu/44992724/Remote_Working_Personality_and_Performance_Research_Results

or work-from-anywhere contexts for some time. Regardless, as leaders, we need to take responsibility for self-leadership while ensuring our members are supported and equipped to be the very best of who they can be. This was my focus.

Of course, going overseas was dependent on the skies remaining open for travel, something that, due to COVID, was not guaranteed. Knowing this, my plan B would allow research to continue; I could still conduct the research through virtual contacts but the key part of having lived experience would be missing.

Obviously, our first choice was to experience first-hand what it meant to work from anywhere and live among cultures not our own. I appreciate this quote from the Interactive Design Foundation (IDF)[10]:

> *"Research can be compared to interacting with the ocean. On the surface, we may see calm beauty or turbulence; however, we can only fully understand the bigger picture once we submerge ourselves and go much deeper. In order to gain a holistic, empathic understanding of [those impacted] and the problem we are trying to solve, we need to question everything, even things that we think we know the answers to."*

There was a certain irony in my undertaking any kind of research. I was never a strong student and lived for the day I would graduate high school and get on with my life. Rather than attending college or university upon graduation, I auditioned for and was accepted into a musical group. The audition was totally unplanned—in fact, I had never even heard of the group before attending their performance that fortuitous night in 1976 in

---

10 "Question Everything," Interactive Design Foundation, accessed April 10,2023, https://www.interaction-design.org/literature/article/question-everything

Niagara Falls, Ontario. Arriving home a few hours later, this seventeen-year-old announced to her parents that she had been accepted into a musical group and needed to be in Florida in a month to begin rehearsals for concerts across the United States in schools, churches, concert halls, and outdoor venues. You can imagine their reaction... a resounding *no*! But, following some investigation into the reputation of the group and a very compelling speech from my older brother, Dad and Mum reconsidered, agreeing that preserving the relationship with their rather impetuous and adventurous daughter was paramount. Four weeks later, I boarded the plane to Orlando, Florida, suitcases filled with myriad costumes my mum and family friend had to sew in preparation for our shows.

Again, the passion for travel served as the impetus for a life-changing decision that found me traversing the United States in a bus for the next two years along with eight fellow singers. I could write a book on the many adventures experienced, but this isn't the place for those stories.

So, how did this non-studious, impetuous, adventurous woman become an academic? You've already read about it back in Chapter 2. What I didn't share is that rather than taking the traditional educational route, after years of industry and leadership experience, at the young age of forty-five, I decided to take a prior learning assessment that, if successful, would allow me to forgo completing an undergrad degree, propelling me into a master's in leadership.

I believe it was Brene Brown that coined the phrase "research storyteller." I like that. Life is full of experiences that call to be shared, and what better way to retell experiences than through stories? My research is built on hearing people's stories, their experiences, and what they learned from those experiences. So, you see, research, to me, isn't about building an academic career. It's about listening, learning, and passing on lessons to others in a way that is practical and applicable. Yes, I have written and published papers on my research, presented on international stages, and been interviewed by podcasters. But more importantly, I've been privileged to sit face-to-face—both physically and virtually—with individuals and teams for the purposes of encouraging, equipping, and co-creating practices with them to help them more effectively lead themselves and their teams. That's what gets me excited! And of course, combining that learning with travel? What's not to love?!

For the next three months, amid our practice trips, I immersed myself in reading books related to leadership, remote work, thinking outside the box, and even deeply philosophical writings that made my brain hurt (see Appendix B). I spoke with more than a hundred folks working in some leadership capacity involving remote and hybrid contexts in various industries. I read relevant publications discovered by my research assistant and analysed them in the context of my research topic. And I blogged—a great way for me to take my research, work through it, and communicate what it meant in practical terms. Honestly, I never imagined how much fun it could be to step away from normal work and focus on this topic. I was truly fortunate. During those times, besides researching, I was also able to present at a virtual conference, work with three companies transitioning to a hybrid model, and coach a leader transitioning to a new career. Working from anywhere *works*. But you need to be well prepared—and open to continued learning.

As I approached this research, my desire was to bracket my own beliefs and adopt a posture of curiosity. One of the first books that stretched my thinking was *Think Again: The Power of Knowing What You Don't Know* by Adam Grant.[11] If you could

---

11 Adam Grant, *Think Again: The Power of Knowing What You Don't Know* (Viking Publishing, 2021).

see the amount of highlights I made in this book, you would grasp the impact it had on my thinking. Here's a quote from the author:

> *"Thinking like a scientist involves more than just reacting with an open mind. It means being actively open-minded. It requires searching for reasons why we might be wrong—not for reasons why we must be right—and revising our views based on what we learn."*

Read that over a few times before moving on... I had to. Let me state again that I am 100 percent Irish, which means I was raised in a home where heated dialogue was welcomed and encouraged, and we learned how to argue our point and get our opinions across before leaving the table. Fairly respectfully, for the most part, but the winner was the one whose idea or opinion was strongest, not the person who was the most open to being wrong. The idea of embarking on research, looking for reasons to prove a hypothesis I had already bought into, was a refreshing concept. Encouraged by Adam Grant, I had to learn how to recognise my cognitive blind spots and revise my thinking accordingly.

In the early stages of the research, I quickly realised the need to ask more questions to gain insight into people's experiences, to intentionally listen hard, to bracket what I thought they might say about how a certain situation could or should have been handled. By learning to think again, I began to watch and listen for the gaps, the pauses, the unspoken emotions—and to gently probe for what was not being said.

As I looked for themes in what it takes to lead in this new context, I began to see that leaders need to be willing to re-think their positions and beliefs, to be OK with admitting they're wrong. I was also more aware of the need for leaders to be willing to provide honest, constructive, specific feedback, even if it wasn't what their members wanted to hear. That takes courage and vulnerability, and a willingness to maybe not win the boss-of-the-month award. It also demonstrates a deep desire to see their team members succeed, and to do what it takes to serve their needs—not those of the leader.

APPENDIX B: BIBLIOGRAPH

Allender, Dan. *Leading with a Limp: Take Full Advantage of Your Most Powerful Weakness.* Waterbrook. 2011.

Buck, John and Eckstein, J. "Changing the culture by changing habits." *Agile Today.* 2019. https://www.agileaus.com.au/changing-the-culture-by-changing-habits/

Coelho, Paulo. *The Alchemist.* Harper One, 1993.

Dam, Rikke Friis, and Siang, Teo Yu. "Question Everything." *Interactive Design Foundation.* https://www.interaction-design.org/literature/article/question-everything

Grant, Adam. *Think Again: The Power of Knowing What You Don't Know.* Viking Publishing, 2021.

Heifetz, R, Grashow, A, and Linsky, M. *The Practice of Adaptive Leadership: Tools and Tactics for Changing Your Organization and the World.* Harvard Business Review Press, 2009.

Lewis, C.S. *Surprised by Joy: The Shape of My Early Life,* HarperOne; Reissue edition, 2017.

MacRea, I. and Sawatzky, R. "Remote Working: Personality and Performance Research Results." *Research Gate* (2020).

Meyer, Erin. *The Culture Map: Breaking Through the Invisible Boundaries of Global Business.* PublicAffairs, 2014.

Scheffler, D. and Guccioine, B. Jr., Loose Canon: The 100 Greatest Travel Books of All Time. *Wonderlust.* https://wonderlusttravel.com/100-greatest-travel-books/.

Sevilla City Office. "Enjoy Flamenco in Seville: Getting to know the soul of a people." Last modified October 2021. https://www.visitasevilla.es/en/history/enjoy-flamencoseville#:~:text=Flamenco%20is%20surely%20the%20purest%20expression%20of%20Andalusian,these%20flamenco%20bars%20opened%20in%20Seville%20around%201885.

"Are You A Sojourner?" *Sojourner Tours*, http://www.sojourner-tours.com/organized-small-group-tour-participant-characteristics.

Strayed, Cheryl. *Wild: From Lost to Found on the Pacific Crest Trail.* Vintage; reprint edition, 2013.

Teresa. "Everything You Need To Know About Las Fallas Festival In Valencia, Spain." *Brogan Abroad.* Last updated February 8, 2023. https://broganabroad.com/fallas-festival-valencia-guide/

APPENDIX C: BOOKS READ FOR RESEARCH

Andreatta, Britt. *Wired to Connect: The Brain Science of Teams and a New Model for Creating Collaboration and Inclusion.* 7th Mind Publishing, 2018.

Banfield, Bart. *Virtual Leadership: The Essential Principles for Remote Work.* Lucid Books, 2020.

Barrett, Frank J. *Yes to the Mess: Surprising Leadership Lessons From Jazz.* Harvard Business Review Press, 2021.

Bolles, Gary A. *The Next Rules of Work: The Mindset, Skill Set and Toolset to Lead Your Organization Through Uncertainty.* 1st ed. Kogan Page, 2021.

Bregman, Rutger. *Humankind: A Hopeful History.* Little, Brown and Company Publishing, 2020.

Dawson, Scott. *The Art of Working Remotely.* 1st ed. Knight Rose Press, 2019.

Eikenberry, K., and W. Turmel. *The Long-Distant Leader: Rules for Remarkable Remote Leadership.* 1st ed. Berrett-Koehler Publishers, 2018.

Elston, John. *The Remote Revolution: How the Location-Independent Workforce Changes the Way We Hire, Connect, and Succeed*. Lioncrest Publishing, 2017.

Eskola, Anne. *Navigating Through Changing Times: Knowledge Work in Complex Environments*. 1st ed. Routledge, 2019.

Fried, J., and D. Heinemeier Hansson. *Remote, Office Not Required*. Currency Publishing, 2013.

Gibbons, Paul. *Impact: 21st Century Change Management Behavioural Science, Digital Transformation and Future of Work*. Phronesis Media Publishing, 2019.

Grant, Adam. *Think Again: The Power of Knowing What You Don't Know*. Viking, 2021.

Gratton, Lynda. *Redesigning Work: How to Transform Your Organization and Make Hybrid Work for Everyone*. MIT Press, 2022.

Hollema, Theresa Sigillito. *Virtual Teams Across Cultures: Create Successful Teams Around The World*. Interact Globa, 2020.

Ivanov, Peter. *Power Teams Beyond Borders: How to Work Remotely and Build Powerful Virtual Teams*. 1st ed. Wiley, 2020.

Jorgan, Jacob. *The Future Leader: 9 Skills and Mindsets to Succeed in the Next Decade*. 1st ed. Wiley, 2020.

Kane, Chris. *Where Is My Office: Reimagining the Workplace for the 21st Century*. Bloomsbury Publishing, 2020.

Kipser, J., and B. Boyd. *Catalyst: Leadership and Strategy in a Changing World*. Lioncrest Publishing, 2018.

Meyer, Erin. *The Culture Map: Breaking Through the Invisible Boundaries of Global Business*. PublicAffairs Publishing, 2016.

Orti, P., and M. Middlemiss. *Thinking Remote: Inspiration for Leaders of Distributed Teams*. Virtual Not Distant, 2019.

Pullan, Penny. *Virtual Leadership: Practical Strategies for Getting the Best Out of Virtual Work and Virtual Teams*. 2nd ed. Kogan, 2022.

Rook, Arthur C. *From Strength to Strength: Finding Success, Happiness and Deep Purpose in the Second Half of Life*. Portfolio Publishing, 2022.

Schawbel, Dan. *Back to Human: How Great Leaders Create Connection in the Age of Isolation*. Da Capo Lifelong Books, 2018.

Swann, Andy. *The Human Workplace: People Centred Organizational Development*. 1st ed. Kogan Page, 2017.

Tierney, V. and Momirov, T. (n.d.) *Your Company with No Walls: How to Master Remote Leadership Fast*.

Withers, Denise. *Story Design: The Creative Way to Innovate*. Produced by Page Two, 2017.

ABOUT THE AUTHOR

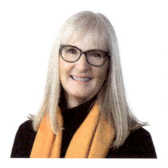

Roberta E. Sawatzky is a business owner, professor, blogger, and avid traveller with a special interest in leadership in remote and hybrid teams. Originally from Bangor, Northern Ireland, travel has always been a major part of her life, with her family taking many sojourns throughout Europe during her youth. Her experience of childhood immigration to Canada would solidify her interest in cross-cultural contact, international travel, and processes of immersion and assimilation. She continued to nurture this interest in both her personal and professional lives, taking many trips for pleasure with family and friends as well as pursuing international research into the characteristics of remote workers, blogging all the while.

When her husband was diagnosed with end-stage renal failure and they were forced to adjust their plans for an extended European trip accordingly, Sawatzky knew she wanted to share their story honestly and openly, providing a vulnerable and inspiring account of their trip. With tenacity and resilience—and perhaps a bit of old-fashioned Irish stubbornness—any challenge, she insists, can be met.

Sawatzky lives with her husband in Kelowna, BC, where together, they enjoy reading, biking, walking, and winery- and café-going. Interested in getting in touch? You can reach her on LinkedIn at linkedin.com/in/robertasawatzky, via email at roberta@samisremote.com or through her business site at www.samisremote.com. You can also read her blogs at probeandponder.com and flexibleworking.blog .

Printed in the USA
CPSIA information can be obtained
at www.ICGtesting.com
LVHW060916301023
762337LV00008B/24